TREE
MEDICINE

'...the leaves of the trees are for the healing of the nations'
Revelation 22

'The Tree is my eternal salvation... Amidst its roots I cast my own roots deep; beneath its boughs I grow and expand; as it sighs around me in the breeze I am nourished with delight.'
St John Chrystomom

TREE MEDICINE

A comprehensive guide to the
healing power of over 170 trees

PETER CONWAY

PIATKUS

For my father

Tree Medicine does not replace normal allopathic medical treatment. It is a means of supporting and complementing such medical treatment. If you have any acute or chronic disease you should seek medical attention from a qualified doctor. The author and publisher accept no liability for damage of any nature resulting directly or indirectly from the application or use of information in this book.

Copyright © 2001 by Peter Conway

First published in 2001 by
Judy Piatkus (Publishers) Limited
5 Windmill Street
London W1T 2JA
e-mail: info@piatkus.co.uk

This paperback edition published in 2002

**For the latest news and information on all our titles
visit our new website at www.piatkus.co.uk**

The moral right of the author has been asserted
A catalogue record for this book is available from the British Library

ISBN 0 7499 2173 0 Hbk
ISBN 0 7499 2273 7 Pbk

Edited by Matthew Cory
Design by Paul Saunders
Botanical illustrations by Lesley Wakerley

This book has been printed on paper manufactured with respect
for the environment using wood from managed sustainable resources

Printed and bound in Great Britain by MPG Books, Bodmin, Cornwall

Contents

Acknowledgements

This book could not have been written without the work of many other people that I have drawn upon for information and inspiration. I would like to thank my colleagues – the traditional and modern healers who keep the practice of plant medicine alive; my teachers, especially Hein Zeylstra, the former Principal of the College of Phytotherapy; the practitioners of ethnobotany; my students; and my patients, who continue to teach and motivate me. Thanks are also due to those who care for the many forests, parks and gardens that have been the main reference works for this book. I am especially grateful to those who founded and continue to run the Royal Botanic Garden, Edinburgh and the Chelsea Physic Garden, London. At Piatkus I am indebted to Sandra Rigby, Claire Richardson, Alice Davis, Matthew Cory and Gill Bailey, but especially to Anne Lawrance – without her vision this book would not have appeared.

Many thanks to Sara Oldfield of the Global Trees Campaign for advising me on the content of chapter 5 on conservation. Any errors are mine, not hers. Much of the information in chapter 5 comes from 'The World List of Threatened Trees' (*see* Bibliography) produced by the World Conservation Monitoring Centre in association with the IUCN, of which Sara was one of the compilers. I would like to gratefully acknowledge this book as a source and pay tribute to the vision and dedication of all those involved in producing it.

The quotes in the section on Art Therapy in Chapter 3 appear by kind permission of *Resurgence* magazine.

I am grateful to Julian Barnard for his advice.

Thank you Kit for your support and wisdom.

Above all, thank you Morgaine, Angelica and Tristan for your patience in giving me time to finish this book.

Introduction

TREES ARE VALUED for many reasons. For their utility in providing us with useful substances such as building materials, fuel, furniture, tools and paper – the tree you are now holding in your hands! For their use in giving us shade and preventing erosion of land. For the foods they give us, mostly their nuts and fruits. For their beauty – they enchant us, inspire us, soothe us and nourish our souls.

But there's more, a further gift that trees bestow upon us – the gift of healing remedies, of medicines. It is surprising that many of us are unaware of this when two of the most widely-used orthodox drugs, aspirin (from willow bark) and chloroquine (a treatment for malaria from Cinchona trees), are derived from trees!

Trees are used in many different types of medicine besides conventional medicine – including herbal medicine, aromatic medicine and aromatherapy, homeopathy and flower remedies. In recent years several books have been written about trees as healing agents from a spiritual–intuitive perspective rather than as sources of medicines. While this book acknowledges the role trees play as a focus in meditation and visualization, it also takes a physical, pharmacologically-based approach to the medicinal properties of trees.

Like most people, I have always had a great fondness for trees. Growing up in the North of England I lived close to Sherwood Forest, the legendary home of Robin Hood, and Clumber Park – one of the great landscaped parks now managed by the National Trust. I remember, as a boy, being taken there for the first time and being deeply moved by the mature trees, awed by their beauty and power. Later, when I trained as a medical herbalist, I learned about the therapeutic value of all types of plants, but I have always retained a particular interest in trees, the monarchs of the plant kingdom. As a herbal practitioner I have seen the ways in which tree medicines have helped my patients recover from a wide variety of diseases and this has led me to extend the range of tree medicines in my practice. I am also a qualified masseur and I have trained in the application of volatile oils (the oils used in aromatherapy) in a therapeutic approach called 'aromatic medicine'. Tree medicines are tremendously versatile and this book looks at all the ways in which we can apply them.

Tree Medicine is divided into two parts. In **Part I** you will find out exactly what tree medicines are, explore the history of the use of trees as sources of remedies, examine the different medical systems that use tree medicines and learn how they can be practically applied. Finally, you will read about the threats to the survival of medicinal trees and the prospects for future developments.

Part II consists of profiles of over 170 individual trees, followed by descriptions of what they have to offer us as remedies.

In the following chapters you will see how trees are an important source of nutritional medicine and learn about tree foods that can boost your immune system, help protect your body from heart disease, and help fight problems such as depression and fatigue. For instance, did you know that Brazil nuts are one of the best sources of the trace mineral selenium and that research shows that eating just one Brazil nut a day can reduce your risk of developing cancer and heart disease, prevent premature ageing, increase fertility in men and reduce the rate of miscarriage in women? Low selenium levels are also associated with depression and other mood disorders. Other nuts have special properties too – almonds are rich in calcium to build healthy bones, hazelnuts have a high zinc content which can improve the function of your immune system and walnuts help to reduce 'bad' cholesterol and increase the amount of healthy HDL cholesterol.

Olive oil is well-known as a dietary aid to decrease cholesterol levels but did you know that studies suggest it can also actually reduce high blood pressure and lessen the need for conventional drugs? The skins of fruits contain pectins that also reduce cholesterol; pectins are a type of soluble fibre that is more effective against cholesterol than bran and much gentler on the digestive system! Everyone knows that fruits contain vitamin C but have you heard of a remarkable South American tree known as camu camu (*Myricaria dubia*) whose fruits are 30 times richer in vitamin C than citrus fruits, making them the most potent source of this important nutrient yet known?

You will also learn about many of the trees used in herbal medicine. These include the extraordinary ginkgo tree, which has been living on the planet for over 180 million years – long before the arrival of human beings. A beautiful deciduous conifer with fan-shaped leaves, an extract from this ancient tree has been shown to aid circulation and is of great benefit in improving concentration, memory and general mental performance. These qualities make it particularly suited to treating degenerative mental disorders in the elderly. Other amazing trees that you will discover include the huge baobab tree (*Adansonia digitata*) that can develop a massive girth and live for over 2,000 years. It is used in Ayurvedic medicine in India for treating fevers, skin disorders and rheumatism. Other long-lived trees are the yews (*Taxus* species) that are used in conventional medicine to treat ovarian and uterine cancers. Several other drugs are being developed from trees to treat serious diseases such as HIV and AIDS.

In considering the history of tree medicines you will read how demand for cloves and nutmeg changed the world! Nutmeg particularly became highly prized in Elizabethan times for its reputation in curing the plague. The English and Dutch East India Companies were founded to secure supplies of the herb and in doing so started the spice trade that helped open up the world to international exploration and exploitation.

One of the great joys for me is the vast breadth of tree medicine and its inclusive, unifying nature linking countries, peoples and cultures all around the world. Each continent has its own unique contributions to make. Within these pages you will find information about trees from many countries and continents, including Africa, Australia, China, Oceania, and South America as well as those from Europe and North America.

The African sausage tree (*Kigelia africana*) has cucumber-shaped fruits that can be made into a cream to treat eczema. Also from Africa are trees (*Acacia* and *Albizzia* species) that the Masai tribe use to prevent their cholesterol saturated diet of milk and blood from causing them severe heart problems. From South America come many valuable tree remedies such as pau d'arco (*Tabebuia* species); these stunning large trees with trumpet-shaped flowers can have a profound effect in enhancing the body's immune system, helping it in fighting infections and other diseases such as cancer.

Australia has many important trees containing volatile oils, such as tea tree (*Melaleuca alternifolia*) which is great for bacterial and fungal infections and several *Eucalyptus* species which have a special role in treating sinus and chest infections. Many European trees are also widely used for their medicinal properties. A very effective cream for varicose veins can be made from the seeds ('conkers') of the horse chestnut tree (*Aesculus hippocastanum*). A delicious calming and relaxing aromatic tea can be made from limeflowers (*Tilia* species) and it also helps to lower blood pressure.

There is one final service that trees give to us, one that is increasingly recognized as being of crucial importance to the whole of life on Earth. Trees provide one of the major environmental control mechanisms for our planet, that of helping to regulate the air we breathe. Trees take in carbon dioxide and give out oxygen, acting as the 'lungs of the planet'; they keep the air clean and healthy. As our modern lifestyles produce greater and greater quantities of carbon dioxide we need this balancing function of trees more than ever. Unfortunately, and most dangerously, while our demand for trees increases the number of trees on earth is diminishing. Deforestation is taking place on a massive scale due to unsustainable harvesting of tree products (including medicines), road building schemes and the demand for farming land. The eventual results of this process are not yet fully understood but the effects of climate change are already being felt and give great cause for concern.

Yet there are many reasons to be optimistic and greater understanding of the significance of trees as vital organs in our world is leading to greater protection of existing populations and also to the planting of new forests. I hope that this book raises awareness of the role of trees as healers to people and that this knowledge will provide support to the movement to conserve and enhance tree populations so that they can continue to fulfil their age-old role of acting as physicians to the planet.

I hope you enjoy your walk through the healing forest.

PETER CONWAY
Edinburgh, February 2001

PART ONE

An Introduction to

Tree

Medicine

1

Planting the Seed –
What is Tree Medicine?

'TREE MEDICINE' is not the latest fashionable complementary therapy; in fact it's not a single therapy at all! As you will see, the medicinal properties of trees are used in several different healing systems including conventional medicine, aromatherapy and homeopathy. While touching on all of these this book focuses on the healing approach that most frequently and most widely uses trees as remedies – herbal medicine.

Some time ago, one of the leading cancer charities launched a poster campaign to raise funds for its research work. One of the slogans they used was 'Cures Don't Grow On Trees' – but they were wrong! Not only do many conventional medicines derive from trees but also several anticancer treatments such as taxol, which was originally found in the Pacific yew tree (*Taxus brevifolia*) and more recently discovered in hazel trees (*Corylus avellana*).

I described herbal medicine as being the main medical system using trees for healing. In the medical sense the word 'herb' means any plant with therapeutic qualities; botanically, though, it refers to a plant whose above ground parts die back each year. While many trees fit the medical definition of herbs, they do not fit the botanical one. So, it might help to start by clarifying what trees actually are.

WHAT IS A TREE?

Trees are the oldest and largest living things on the planet. The majority of trees live for hundreds of years. Birches (*Betula* species) live for 80–200 years, beech (*Fagus sylvatica*) 200–400 years, and Scots pine for around 500 years. But some trees live even longer – oaks (*Quercus* species) can make around 1,000 years, coastal redwoods (*Sequoia sempervirens*) over 2,000 and giant sequoias (*Sequoiadendron giganteum*) over 3,000 years. Amongst the oldest living trees on the planet are the North American bristle-cone pines (*Pinus aristata*) – one has been dated at over 4,600 years old. Even these are eclipsed by the European yew tree (*Taxus baccata*) that can live for well over 5,000 years, although yew trees are hard to date.

The age of trees is calculated by counting their rings but yews often become hollow in the centre as they age and this destroys much of the evidence! Also, they can grow to a huge girth making it difficult to obtain a core sample (chopping down an ancient tree to count its rings is, thankfully, deemed unethical!). A remarkable yew tree in a churchyard in the small Scottish village of Fortingall has been dated by the Forestry Commission as being over 8,000 years old. This is considered to be the oldest tree in Europe. Local legend has it that Pontius Pilate was born in the Roman encampment just by this marvellous tree, and he may have played in it as a boy.

Yews are also amongst the widest trees. The Fortingall yew once had a diameter of 5.4m (17ft 8in). Giant sequoias, baobabs (*Adansonia digitata*), oaks, sweet chestnuts and limes can all achieve impressive girths. The extraordinary banyan trees (*Ficus benghalensis*) increase their size by sending out roots from their branches. The above ground portions of the roots appear to be 'trunks' as they provide support for the tree to develop its girth. Such trees can cover huge areas, potentially extending over several acres! In terms of height the coastal redwoods are the recorded champions, the largest measured example coming in at 112.2m (368ft). Certain eucalyptus species and Douglas firs (*Pseudotsuga* species) are said to grow even taller.

So, trees can live for a long time and they can be very big, but we really need a more precise definition – for instance what is the difference between a tree and a shrub? There is no single agreed definition of what constitutes a tree but in general we can say that *a tree has a single self-supporting perennial woody stem that branches at some distance from the ground.*

Shrubs, by contrast, have several stems coming directly up from the ground and are usually smaller than trees. However, the distinction is not always clear. For example, the elder (*Sambucus nigra*) may develop as a shrub or as a tree depending on its growing conditions. For our purposes I have tried to stick to the strict definition of a tree but some of the plants included are described as being 'a shrub or small tree' to reflect the overlap that frequently occurs. I have also excluded palms as it has been argued that they are not trees at all. Also not included are the many plants that grow in conjunction with trees, such as vines, lianas, mistletoe and those herbaceous plants that grow in woods and forest and depend on tree shade.

Before moving on it will help to understand how the different types of trees are classified and to learn some of the words used to describe trees. The main botanical division is based on how the seeds are presented on the tree. Trees are placed within one of two groups:

GYMNOSPERMS – trees that have 'naked seeds', displayed to the air and visible to the eye;

ANGIOSPERMS – trees whose seeds are hidden within a fruit.

The gymnosperm group is largely made up of the conifers such as pine trees. The angiosperms are further divided (again according to the seed type) as **monocotyledons** (seeds having just one embryonic leaf) and **dicotyledons** (seeds having two embryonic leaves). Most angiosperm trees are contained within the dicotyledon group.

Many of the words used to classify trees further can be a little confusing and need to be explained, these include:

SOFTWOOD and HARDWOOD – these terms are used by the timber industry to describe trees based on the density of their wood. Gymnosperms are said to possess soft wood and angiosperms to have hard wood. While it is true that the wood of one group tends to be soft and that of the other to be hard there are exceptions. For instance, balsa wood (*Ochroma pyramidale*) used in modelling (for instance, children's toy aeroplanes) comes from the hardwood group. Yew, one of the hardest of woods, is placed within the softwood group.

EVERGREENS and DECIDUOUS – evergreen trees keep their leaves all year round whereas deciduous trees lose theirs once a year. The gymnosperms are thought of as being evergreens while the angiosperms are said to be deciduous. However this is not always the case; some gymnosperms (such as *Ginkgo biloba*) are in fact deciduous and some angiosperms (such as the holm oak – *Quercus ilex*) are evergreen. Also, the tendency to be deciduous in angiosperms depends largely on climate – if grown in tropical climes many of these trees can take on an evergreen habit.

NEEDLES and **BROADLEAVES** – many gymnosperms have needles but some have scaly leaves (such as cypress trees – *Cupressus* species) and others have broadleaves.

WHAT IS A MEDICINE?

Having established what a tree is you should also understand what is meant by the term 'medicine'; what do we consider as being the healing properties of trees? A broad holistic view of a medicine might be that *a medicine is any substance that tends to promote health and well-being, prevent illness and/or treat disease.*

We tend to view only the latter aspect, the treatment of disease, as being the role of a medicine but the promotion of health and well-being and the prevention of illness are arguably of more importance. If we lead healthy and contented lives then we are less likely to become unwell. Prevention is always better than cure. While some conditions, notably genetically inherited disorders, may not be preventable, many others (in fact, the majority of illnesses) are. Trees are valuable in promoting health and preventing disease in various ways, including:

- **stress reduction** – trees such as lime (*Tilia* species) have relaxing and calming effects that help to reduce the impacts of stress on our bodies;

- **immune boosting** – elderberries are one example of tree products that can help improve our resistance to disease;

- **regulation of digestion** – good digestive functioning is essential for health. Tree medicines can improve the way we digest and absorb foods (such as quassia – *Picrasma excelsa*) and regulate bowel movements whether there is constipation (such as cascara sagrada – *Rhamnus purshiana*) or looseness of the motions (such as rowan berries – *Sorbus aucuparia*);

- **nutrition** – perhaps most importantly of all, trees have a major role to play in providing a healthy diet. Consumption of olive oil helps to keep cholesterol levels low. Tree fruits such as peaches, apricots and apples provide us with powerful antioxidants that can help prevent heart disease and some cancers.

Essentially we have four levels of activity as human beings and we can experience wellness or illness on all these levels. They are:

- the physical level;

- the emotional level;

- the mental level;

- the spiritual level.

As individuals we may be focused on one level more than others at particular times in our lives. If we are studying for examinations we are working mainly on the mental level. Following bereavement we tend to be hit most deeply at the emotional level, often then moving on to seek understanding at the spiritual level.

While no one inhabits any one particular level exclusively many of us lean towards one aspect rather than another. Athletes concentrate on the physical (though they have to overcome their emotional anxieties and achieve mental control if they are to succeed); religious leaders focus on the spiritual (yet they must stay rooted to the physical world if their activities are to benefit humanity). As we grow we tend to move through the levels – from relating to the world physically as a child, through the emotional times of adolescence, achieving greater mental control and knowledge as we mature and finally reaching a more contemplative spiritual outlook in old age. Tree medicines relate to these levels in a number of ways:

- **physical** – the nutritional content of tree fruits helps to build a strong and resilient body. Trees can treat physical problems such as wounds (for instance, witch hazel – *Hamamelis virginiana*) and pain (such as cloves – *Syzygium aromaticum* – for toothache);

- **emotional** – trees can promote emotional stability by regular use of teas such as limeflower, and treat mood disorders such as anxiety (for example, Jamaican dogwood – *Piscidia erythrina*) and depression (such as neroli oil – *Citrus aurantium*);

- **mental** – the leaves of *Ginkgo biloba* promote blood circulation to the brain and improve concentration and memory skills;

- **spiritual** – this is an area where less is really known about the effects of medicinal substances. Spending time in the company of trees can have a very nourishing and supportive effect, helping to lift our spirits and inspire us.

You can now see that trees can have an influence on every level of our being and can play an important part in helping us to maintain optimum health. However, there are times when prevention fails and illness becomes established. When sickness is present, tree medicines can be used in a number of ways depending on the type of condition. In severe illnesses treatment is often required in hospital and this might include the use of a conventional pharmaceutical medicine derived from a tree, such as taxol for treating cancer. For many mild to moderate conditions several types of tree medicines are available.

Tree medicine is not a systematic therapy in itself, rather trees are made use of as an element in several healing systems. The differences in the way the trees are employed as healing agents are explained in more detail in chapter 4.

The manner in which trees are prepared for use across the many therapies also varies widely. Various parts of the trees are processed to form a number of different preparations, including the use of whole leaves and berries in herbal medicine; the pressed oils applied to the skin in massage and the distilled volatile (essential) oils that form the main tools of aromatherapy; and the highly purified (and often artificially synthesized) compounds given as conventional drugs. In some cases the trees are not made into preparations at all. They are used 'as they are', as in art therapy and when used as a focus for meditation.

'Healing gardens' also have great potential to help patients recovering from illness. Hospitals and health centres may incorporate gardens as places of sanctuary and inspiration and such buildings can be planned around gardens in order that patients can overlook trees and other plants from the windows. Patients who are well enough are able to go outside and sit with trees, drawing strength from them. To see fruit trees in blossom, birches turning golden at autumn time, to hear the wind given a voice by a myriad of leaves and to smell earthy bark or ethereal flowers – these are all stimulants to the soul that can support rejuvenation of the body.

Nature can offer her gifts even in terminal illness. I recall watching the playwright Dennis Potter being interviewed as he was dying from cancer. He spoke about the tremendous comfort that contemplation of the beauty of blossom had brought him and how he wished he had spent more of his life enjoying such experiences.

The Scope of Tree Medicine

To help understand the breadth of the healing contribution that trees can make it is useful to look at the range of diseases themselves. They can be viewed as covering a spectrum ranging from **preventable**, through **mild**, **moderate** and **severe**, to **terminal**.

At the preventable end of the spectrum, antioxidants from tree fruits (such as cherries and mulberries) can help prevent cancer and heart disease. The use of tree foods, such as fruits and nuts, can help correct nutritional deficiencies and help to restore the body to health during periods of stress and during convalescence following illness. They may also help prevent more serious disease from developing. Selenium, a nutrient obtained most readily from Brazil nuts (the seeds of the giant rainforest tree *Betholletia excelsa*), is vital to maintain healthy nerve function – deficiency can lead to depression and infertility. The lack of specific nutrients can be linked to numerous general symptoms such as fatigue, decreased concentration, skin disorders and irritability. In terms of prevention of disease, tree nutrients have a major protective role to play.

Different illnesses can vary from being mild to severe. Conditions such as eczema and acne may be described as mild in some cases. A small patch of non-irritating eczema on the arms can be largely forgotten about because it causes little disruption to living our daily lives. But, if the eczema is more widespread, itchy or weeping, and on the hands or face, it can cause moderate to severe problems. Marked itchiness should be viewed as a form of pain since it can cause great suffering. To those not afflicted by acne, this may seem to be a mild disease but, when it is pronounced, it can hugely affect the sufferer's self-confidence. Persons with acne may have low self-esteem, avoid social situations and develop deep depression – this is a severe state to be in.

Severe illness includes many conditions that may require treatment in hospital. Such problems include ulcerative colitis and Crohn's disease, multiple sclerosis, and severe infections like pneumonia. Even here there are variations. For example, while ulcerative colitis can be an extreme problem at times, there are also periods where it only affects the sufferer to a mild extent. Many severe illnesses can be life-threatening at times, though they are not always inevitably so. Pneumonia is a major cause of death, particularly in the elderly, but with swift treatment and the best care it may often be treated successfully. With regard to terminal illness, there often comes a point when both the person and their carers realize that it has become inappropriate to continue to fight and the emphasis moves to promoting the person's comfort and contentment. Here the less directly physical tree therapies can have a significant role – to lift the spirits and accompany the soul as it prepares for its journey beyond the body.

Trees, of course, do not hold the answer to all problems, but they do constitute a huge natural medicine chest. They provide substances that can be used alongside other treatment options to help improve many health difficulties. In Part II of this book you will find profiles of over 170 medicinal trees that between them can help with a vast array of medical conditions.

As we move from one end of the illness spectrum to the other, the types of tree preparation that we use can change. At the preventable level we are mainly using trees in their gentlest form – as foods. As we progress to mild and severe disease we are principally using appropriate herbal medicine preparations. At the severe to terminal end of the spectrum conventional drugs prepared from trees play an increasing role. As the degree of disease increases we often need to respond with stronger and stronger tree preparations. This leads us into questioning the safety of tree medicines. How safe are they and what risks do they carry?

ARE TREE MEDICINES SAFE?

People tend to use complementary medicines because they believe them to be safer than conventional medicines. It is certainly the case that most alternative remedies do appear to be safer than most conventional drugs but this isn't a hard and fast rule. In the literature accompanying their drugs all pharmaceutical manufacturers are obliged to list all the potential side effects their products can cause. This does not mean that every person taking each drug will experience every listed side effect – far from it. Many drugs, when appropriately prescribed and correctly monitored, have more good than bad effects. This is known as the risk–benefit ratio.

All drugs should have positive effects that outweigh any negative effects that may accompany them. For example, the source of quinine, Peruvian bark (*Cinchona* species), can be valuable in malaria and fevers but it can also cause a syndrome known as cinchonism that causes headaches, abdominal pains and disturbances in hearing and vision. Some trees need to be avoided in specific situations, such as during pregnancy, and others are so toxic that they should always be avoided completely. One example of the latter type of tree is *Croton tiglium* that yields croton oil – this is one of the most drastically purgative (causing severe diarrhoea and vomiting) substances known.

Just as there is a spectrum of disease, tree preparations spread across a spectrum of safety. This extends from **safe** to **gentle, intermediate** and **strong,** to **toxic.**

Tree medicines at the safe end are those that appear to be completely well tolerated causing no known side effects. In this group are the healing foods such as olive oil, prunes, apples and hazelnuts. Almost everyone can take these tree products as part of a varied healthy diet and they can help prevent or treat certain conditions such as lowered immune resistance or fatigue. The gentle remedies are those that are considered specifically as medicines rather than, or as well as being, foods and which have a reputation for being virtually free of side effects. Trees in this category include spices such as star anise (*Illicium verum*) and cinnamon bark (*Cinnamomum zeylanicum*), as well as elderflowers (*Sambucus nigra*) and limeflowers (*Tilia* species). Some minor side effects may occur – for example limeflowers are gently soothing and calming to the nervous system but they may prove actively sedating in persons with depleted energy levels causing them to experience fatigue.

Trees in the intermediate category are generally well tolerated but may cause side effects that raise more concern if used without due caution. An example of this is the spindle tree (*Euonymus purpurea*) – the bark is useful as a stimulant to the liver and gallbladder but it can cause marked digestive upsets with vomiting and diarrhoea. Strong tree medicines are those that tend to have very pronounced effects on bodily functions, are prone to triggering significant side effects, and may exacerbate certain medical conditions. An example of this is yohimbe (*Pausinystalia johimbe*) which is used to treat impotence and is an effective aphrodisiac, but it can also cause severe headaches and psychiatric disorders, and can worsen high blood pressure.

Trees in the toxic category should only be used when there is an overwhelming good reason to do so. Many of the conventional drugs derived from trees fall within this category. Such tree medicines may offer benefits but only in very particular circumstances and only when used with the very greatest of care.

Generally, the trees in the safe or gentle groups are suitable for home use on a self-prescribed basis by most people. Those in the intermediate to toxic categories should only be taken following expert professional advice.

Another factor to consider is the potential for adverse reactions occurring between natural medicines and conventional drugs. This is something of a grey area and it is now receiving closer scrutiny as complementary medicines are more frequently taken in conjunction with orthodox drugs. It is often possible to take safe and gentle tree medicines with many drugs without any problems occurring. However, it is always advisable to inform your doctor of any natural medicines you are taking. There are only a few clear examples where herbal tree medicines should definitely be avoided with certain drugs; these include *Ginkgo biloba* that should not be taken alongside blood thinning (anticoagulant drugs) such as warfarin.

As a general rule, the more you purify a medicine the greater becomes its potential to cause side effects. Herbal medicines are minimally processed (at their simplest, dried plant parts are simply infused in hot water) and contain hundreds of different chemicals. This diversity tends to include substances that balance the plant's action, preventing it from acting in too strong a manner.

Volatile (essential) oils used in aromatherapy are extracts of a particular group of plant chemicals. These oils are still quite chemically diverse but far less so than herbal medicines. So, they are more likely to cause problems and should not be taken by mouth or applied neat to the skin unless on expert professional advice.

Conventional drugs are highly purified and contain just one or two distinct chemicals. Such pure chemicals can often have rapid and pro-nounced beneficial effects but are unchecked by balancing cofactors and have the highest potential to cause problems.

The conventional pharmacological wisdom is that any substance that has the capacity to heal also possesses the potential to harm. Advocates of complementary medicine stress that one of the main benefits of their treatment is its strong safety profile. It is important to remember, though, that a medicine is not automatically safe just because it is natural. Tree medicines of all types can be powerful healing agents and should be treated with respect. If you are in any doubt as to how to proceed with a tree medicine, or if your condition does not respond to treatment or it worsens – always consult an expert.

USING TREE MEDICINES

There are several ways in which you can use trees to improve your health. One option is to consult a herbal practitioner for treatment when health problems arise. But there are a variety of other different medical systems that use trees to treat particular conditions and these are described in detail in chapter 4. However, there are ways by which you can make the healing power of trees part of your daily life.

Trees in your diet

To harness the preventive medicine effects of trees by using them as foods is easy and delicious! The main tree foods are nuts and fruits – as well as being delightful to eat they possess many healthy properties. Below are some suggestions for incorporating the benefits of trees as part of your normal diet. For further information, turn to the section on nutritional medicine in Chapter 4.

Nuts

Nuts contain important essential fatty acids and a wide range of nutrients including protein, B vitamins and vitamin E. Almonds are a good source of calcium. Brazil nuts, almonds, walnuts and hazelnuts are good providers of zinc that is important for optimum functioning of the immune system, skin health and wound healing. Brazil nuts are a prime source of selenium. Walnuts and hazelnuts contain useful amounts of folic acid.

Nuts can be taken at breakfast time in home-made muesli – mixing nuts, dried fruits, seeds and oats. Muesli is often more palatable if you soak it overnight and add a little fresh fruit in the morning. It is good to use nuts as a substitute for snack foods such as crisps and sweets. Keep a bag of mixed nuts in your bag or in a drawer at work so they are to hand when you need them.

Nuts can be made into butters as an alternative to peanut butter by blending them with oil and a little salt. Hazelnut, almond and cashew butters are available commercially and they are often very popular with children. Sweet chestnuts are wonderful when roasted. Beech nuts are not often available for sale but are worth collecting from the wild, they have a crisp texture and are very tasty.

Fruits

Tree fruits can be taken fresh or dried. Fruits contain a number of important nutrients including vitamin C, beta-carotene, minerals and trace minerals such as boron (which is helpful in supporting healthy bone and joint functioning). Uncooked fruits keep their vitamin content better than cooked fruits. Dried fruits contain complex sugars that are slowly released into the body so that they give a sustained energy release, avoiding the peaks and troughs caused by purified sugars. This means that dried fruit is a good snack food as a replacement for confectionery. Keep some dried fruit in your bag as you travel. It also makes a good sweet treat for children as an alternative to other snacks – dried pears and apples are particular favourites. Dried apricots, prunes and figs are rich in iron. Figs are also a good calcium source. Dried apricots are good for women during menstruation; they can also help control the low blood sugar levels that some women get before their periods causing fatigue, irritability and food cravings. The sugars in fruit do not cause tooth decay, unless the fruit has been processed, for example into prepared fruit juices.

Fruit has potent antioxidant effects that protect the body's cells from damage and can help prevent serious disease and boost the immune system. Chemical compounds based on flavonoids have these beneficial properties. It is recommended that we all eat 5–6 portions of fruit/vegetables each day. Try to eat 3 pieces of fruit a day, get into the habit of snacking on fruit rather than fatty or sugary convenience foods. This will help you to avoid heart disease and to improve your defence mechanisms. People who eat fruit regularly tend to find they experience fewer winter coughs and colds.

One of the easiest and most useful ways to enjoy fruits is to make fruit salads. For those people who find it difficult to tolerate much fruit, try cutting several fruits up into a manageable size, mixing them together and adding freshly squeezed fruit juice. Organic fruit is preferable as non-organic fruit may contain harmful chemical residues. (It is sensible to peel all non-organic fruit before eating.) Fruit peel is important, though, as it contains pectins, which are a type of soluble fibre. Pectins help to engender normal healthy bowel movements and lower cholesterol levels.

Trees in Your Kitchen

Trees can be used as ingredients in cooking in so many ways. Spices such as cloves, cinnamon and allspice can be used in sweet and savoury dishes. Oils such as olive, hazelnut and walnut add exciting variations in taste. Olives themselves are widely used. Olive pâté (olives blended with olive oil and flavourings such as chilli peppers) makes a wonderful nutritious and satisfying sandwich spread or dip. Another dip is guacamole which is based on avocados. Avocados contain vitamin E and important essential fatty acids and they encourage healthy skin and hair growth.

One of the best ways to enjoy the benefits of trees in the diet is to make salad dressings that can be used to provide a regular nutritional supplement of beneficial oils, vitamin C, enzymes, antioxidants and antiseptic volatile oils; as in the following recipe.

> Cold pressed extra virgin olive oil – 200ml (7 fl oz)
> Cider apple vinegar – 50ml (2 fl oz)
> Freshly squeezed lemon juice – 50ml (2 fl oz)
> 2–3 bay (*Laurus nobilis*) leaves
>
> Combine the ingredients in a bottle. Crush the bay leaves (by going over them with a rolling pin) before adding. Shake well and set aside for the bay leaves to slowly infuse into the oil. Shake again each time before using.

This dressing can be taken regularly, poured on salads, to promote optimum health.

Teas

The main beverages consumed in the Western world are tea (China or Indian tea) and coffee. Tea and coffee are not included in the tree profiles part of this book as they are shrubs rather than trees. Green tea is becoming increasingly popular since it is a potent source of antioxidants. Black tea also contains some antioxidants but it also has several downsides. It is a moderate nervous stimulant and can cause irritability and interfere with blood sugar control. The tannins in tea can bind to essential nutrients such as iron and prevent their proper absorption. Heavy tea drinking can be linked with nutritional deficiencies. Coffee is another stimulant that can cause anxiety, panic attacks, headaches, irritability and insomnia.

Cocoa is a popular beverage made from the pods of the tree *Theobroma cacao*. Although *Theobroma* translates as 'the food of the gods' it will not suit mere mortals who suffer from migraines as cocoa can trigger off these severe headaches. Fortunately there are other herbal teas from trees that can offer healthy alternatives. Carob (*Ceratonia siliqua*) is a good substitute for cocoa, having a similar colour, texture and taste but being gentle and non-stimulating. (The best substitute for tea is the South African shrub *Aspalanthus linearis*, called rooibosch or red bush. This is rich in antioxidants, non-stimulating, low in tannins and absolutely delicious).

With herbal teas from trees, you can move beyond the tea, coffee, chocolate trinity into a wider world of healthy and enjoyable beverages.

As an example, try this relaxing and calming tea at the end of the day to help you unwind. (Do not use it if you are suffering from pronounced fatigue or low blood pressure.)

Crataegus species (hawthorn) leaves and flowers – 1 teaspoon (2g)
Viburnum prunifolium (black haw) bark – ½ teaspoon (2g)
Tilia europaea (limeflowers) – 1 teaspoon (2g)

Pour 250ml (a mugful) of just boiled water over the herbs, cover over and leave to brew for 5 minutes, then stir, strain and drink. Take this tea 2–3 times a day, in the afternoon and evening.

There are more tea recipes in **Tree Profiles** in Part II of this book. You can obtain teabags of individual herbs such as limeflowers or elderflowers. These are ideal for using when at work or when you don't have time to make a loose herb tea. For full details on tea preparation, *see* Chapter 4.

Trees as Cosmetics

A number of trees are used in the manufacture of cosmetic products. French olive oil soap comes in wonderful big green squares and helps to leave the skin sleek and healthy looking. Several tree volatile oils are added to cleaning preparations as scents and antiseptics. Ylang ylang (*Cananga odorata*) is popular in soaps for its flowery perfume. Pine oil is favoured as a rugged 'manly' scent and it makes an effective ingredient in relaxing bath products.

Tea tree is found in everything from shampoos to shower gels where it can be of particular benefit if you suffer from fungal skin infections. A word of caution though, tea tree is quite drying to the skin and may cause allergic skin reactions if the concentration of the oil in the product is high.

Quassia (*Picrasma excelsa*) shampoo is valuable in treating head lice, it is much safer than conventional drug alternatives and can be used repeatedly for children without causing any ill effects. Distilled witch hazel (*Hamamelis virginiana*) water is well-known and widely used as a make-up remover. It is also cooling and soothing to slight burns, grazes and insect bites. Conkers, the fruit of the beautiful horse chestnut tree (*Aesculus hippocastanum*), provide an important skin treatment. A constituent called aescin has strengthening effects on skin cells making horse chestnut creams useful in improving poor skin tone, treating cellulite and even helping to prevent the effects of skin ageing. Another interesting skin product is an extract from the sap of the sugar maple (*Acer saccharum*). This is applied as a nourishing skin moisturiser.

Trees for Your Spirit

Trees can enhance our emotional, mental and spiritual aspects, as well as the physical. We can gain nourishment from trees on these levels in a number of ways. It is likely you already have trees growing in your garden or near to where you live. Take time to get to know your local trees better. Learn their names. Explore the trees that you feel drawn to. Spend time observing them – how do they strike you, how do they make you feel? Each tree is a living thing, an individual; each has its own unique qualities. You can come closer to trees by simply sitting with them, or you could try to sketch or paint them, take a photograph, or even write a poem about them. Children love to do all these things with trees. They also like to use paper and crayons to take bark rubbings, and to collect an assortment of leaves and do rubbings of them as well. Trees make very good company! Whenever possible carry out your everyday activities, such as working, reading and eating, close to trees. Their calming influence will gently seep in to you and promote a sense of well-being.

If you have enough space then plant some trees. You don't need a lot of room – fruit trees can be trained against a wall, taking up almost no space at all! Some trees will grow well in pots so you can grow them even if you only have a small balcony to put them on! Think about which trees you want to plant, what do you want from them – fruit, nuts, medicines, shade, autumn colour, scent? Find out how big the tree will grow, does it have enough sun or shade? Choosing and planting a tree, then watching it grow can be a very rewarding experience. There is an extra dimension when the tree is planted to mark a significant event – such as a birth or death.

It is great to get out and visit woods, forests, parks and gardens. Different localities and collections have different things to offer. Trees are so prevalent in many areas that sometimes we forget about them. The key is just to become more aware of what is already around us. Look out for the trees in your locality, tune into them – they will repay your attention.

The Tree Remedy box

It is worth keeping a few key tree medicines near to hand in case of emergencies. You could add these to a first aid box or keep a separate collection in a special place. In my practice I have several wooden boxes where I store groups of remedies, for example I have one made of storm-damaged yew where I keep several of my volatile oils.

A good starter tree medicine collection might include the following:

TREE MEDICINE REMEDY BOX

- tea tree (*Melaleuca alternifolia*) volatile oil – for skin infections;

- eucalyptus volatile oil – to make a chest rub and inhalation for coughs, blocked sinuses and chest infections;

- myrrh (*Commiphora molmol*) tincture – to use as a gargle for throat infections;

- slippery elm (*Ulmus rubra*) powder – to make into a paste as a 'drawing cream' to remove splinters and thorns from the skin;

- pine (*Pinus* species) volatile oil – to add to baths to stimulate circulation when you have caught a chill, and to massage into stiff muscles;

- witch hazel (*Hamamelis virginiana*) bark tincture – to apply to small cuts to stop bleeding;

- dried clove (*Syzygium aromaticum*) buds – to treat toothache and ease digestive spasms;

- black haw (*Viburnum prunifolium*) tincture – for when there is severe muscular tension;

- dried elderflowers (*Sambucus nigra*) – to make into a tea at the first sign of colds and flu;

- Jamaica dogwood (*Piscidia erythrina*) tincture – to take to calm anxiety and nervous tension and help with insomnia.

You might also want to include some of the Bach Flower Remedies such as cherry plum (for when there is great fear), olive (for exhaustion) and crab apple (for cleansing).

2

Putting Down Roots –
A Brief History of Trees
in Medicine

THE FIRST TREES appeared on this planet some 390 million years ago. Most of the early species are now extinct, perishing for many reasons including their destruction in the Ice Age. One ancient survivor is the ginkgo tree (*Ginkgo biloba*). Not only is it the oldest tree species on the planet, it may be the single most important medicinal tree we have. *Ginkgo biloba* can trace its origin back around 180 million years, long before the appearance of human beings. The species *biloba* (so named because ginkgo leaves are fan shaped and often have a deep fissure in the centre dividing the leaf into two (*bi-*) distinct sections or lobes (-*loba*)) is the last surviving member of the Ginkgo family. It is likely that it has only endured due to human cultivation, being kept alive because it was valued as a source of food, wood, and medicine and also for its great beauty. Its ability to persist is symbolized by its involvement in one of the twentieth century's most dramatic events. On 6 August 1945 the first atomic bomb was dropped on Hiroshima, the wave of almost total destruction spread over several miles. From this huge field of obliteration one tree, near the epicentre of the blast, managed to regenerate itself – a ginkgo tree.

Trees such as ginkgo pre-date the presence of human beings; they existed way before the concept of 'medicine' was formulated. So how have we developed our knowledge of the healing properties of these plants? The answer is that, since the understanding of the therapeutic qualities of many plants extends into prehistory, we simply cannot be sure. It is likely that most awareness came about through happy accident, or trial and error.

There are other theories about how our first knowledge came about. One such is that our early ancestors had a kind of instinctual knowledge of plant medicines much as some animals appear to have today. Both wild and domesticated animals seem to have some knowledge of which plants to eat when they are ill – they appear to know, to a limited extent, how to self-medicate with specific herbs for certain conditions. Another theory that has been popular is that of the 'doctrine of signatures'. This holds that there is something about a plant's physical characteristics that can reveal its medicinal properties to the sensitive investigator. In many ways this is a mystical religious idea that God has somehow created a sign of the plant's value for the enlightened person to recognize. Such a sign might pertain to the plant's growing habit, its colour, smell, shape or other features. For example, the willow (*Salix* species) has traditionally been used to treat stiff and painful joints. According to the doctrine of signatures, the properties of willow are signed by the ability of willow trees to bend in the wind, to move with ease, by their suppleness and ability to flex without breaking. In addition, willows favour growing in damp places – the symptoms of arthritis and rheumatism are often exacerbated by damp atmospheres. It could be that the concept of the doctrine of signatures is a corruption of the learning methods of the oral tradition. Before written records were common, knowledge was passed on by word of mouth and the 'sign' was used as a mnemonic device to aid learning.

PLANTS AND HUMAN HISTORY

The history of humanity can be seen, in one sense, as the history of our relationship with plants. Without plants we could not live at all. We depend on them for food; they are important for building our homes and, at certain points in history, trees have played the hugely significant role of providing the materials for making ocean-going ships. The international travel this facilitated is arguably the single most important catalyst for change in human history – bringing as it did the dissemination of catastrophic disease, epidemics and massive cultural upheavals. Plagues and other diseases were spread around the world by sea travel and the introduction of these diseases often had catastrophic consequences such as when the Spanish conquistadors brought Old World infections to South America. The worldwide trade made possible by ocean-going ships brought cultures into contact as never before and often led to battles and wars as well as the beneficial exchange of goods and information.

Mythology and legend attest to the central role that trees have occupied as symbols. Most cultures have a variation on the theme of the 'tree of life', from the tree in the Garden of Eden to Yggdrasill, the sacred World Tree of Norse mythology. Certain varieties of tree are seen as sacred by numerous cultures. In India, banyan (*Ficus benghalensis*), fig (*Ficus carica*) and neem (*Azadirachta indica*) have long been revered by the Hindus. The oil from sandalwood (*Santalum album*) remains an important element of Hindu religious ceremonies just as frankincense (*Boswella sacra*) and myrrh (*Commiphora molmol*) in the Christian traditions. Trees were crucial elements in the world of the Druids of ancient Britain. The word Druid itself derives from *dru*, meaning oak, and *druidh* – truth. Early Celtic peoples made use of a tree alphabet called ogham.

Specific individual trees have been revered throughout time and all over the planet. One that I am particularly familiar with is the Glastonbury thorn (*Crataegus monogyna* cv. Biflora). Legend has it that Joseph of Arimathea sailed to England following the death of Jesus Christ and upon arrival stuck his staff into the ground on top of Wearyall Hill within the bounds of Glastonbury. The staff then burst into flower and remained rooted to the hill. At some point the original tree was cut down but parts of it grow in nearby Glastonbury Abbey on what is known as 'the holyest erthe in Englande'.

In many countries individual trees are seen as bringing good luck and are known as 'wish trees'. The tree's luck may be sought by touching it or tying a piece of cloth to it. I remember being taken to a wish tree in Ireland as a child. The goodwill of this tree was obtained by hammering a coin into it as you made your wish. It was an amazing sight, a huge old tree glittering with coins! Other specific trees have been seen as having healing properties with sick people being passed through clefts in them, being associated with fertility, or containing demons or the souls of the dead.

In many cultures all trees have been held as sacred, the idea being that each tree is inhabited by a spirit that may be benevolent if treated with due respect. The ancient writer Porphyry wrote:

They say that primitive man led an unhappy life, for their superstition did not stop at animals but extended even to plants. For why should the slaughter of an ox or a sheep be a greater wrong than the felling of a fir or an oak, seeing that a soul is implanted in these trees also?

A more direct expression of the intimate relationship with trees is given by the Native American Tatanga Mani, or Walking Buffalo, who, when aged 87, said the following during a lecture in London in 1958:

Did you know that trees talk? Well they do. They talk to each other, and they'll talk to you if you listen… I have learned a lot from trees: sometimes about the weather, sometimes about animals, sometimes about the Great Spirit.

One important way that this dialogue with trees, and indeed all plants, has been facilitated in a healing sense has been through the practices of the shaman. Shamans are traditional healers who journey to the spirit world to communicate with plants, animals, rocks and ancestors in order to diagnose disease, draw down healing energy and seek advice about treatment. Underlying the shamans' activities is a core belief in the sentience and wisdom of nature.

The key tools that make the shamans' spiritual journeys possible are hallucinogenic plants such as peyote cactus (*Lophophora williamsii*) in North America and the ayahuasca vine (*Banisteriopsis caapi*) in South America. Among the most important trees used as hallucinogens in South America are the *Virola* species, members of the nutmeg family. The inner bark of the tree is prepared for use and is either taken by mouth or as a snuff blown into the shaman's nose through a tube by an assistant. The psychoactive tryptamines in the tree act quickly to produce visions and connect the shaman with the spirit world. The shaman will then try and track down the cause of the patient's illness – often literally – employing the aid of animal guides that help to locate the illness as a 'prey' that can be killed, and the patient therefore healed, during the shaman's journey. Alternatively, plant spirits may indicate the type of herbs that the patient needs to be given.

However one views the value of shamanic practices, it is important to be aware that this kind of healing, made possible by powerful plant hallucinogens, has been one of the major healing strategies of humanity over very many years. From a modern scientific perspective, the least we can say is that the sight of the shaman working under the influence of hallucinogenic herbs makes a powerful impression on the patient and that this, coupled with the patient's strong belief in the healing power of the shaman, creates a placebo effect that rallies the patient's own innate self-healing abilities.

Our knowledge of shamanism is based on the work of researchers who have collected material on this subject from what is a largely oral tradition. However, there are a number of important written texts that give us an insight into how trees were used in ancient medicine. One of the earliest of these is the Chinese 'Divine Husbandsman's Classic of the Materia Medica' (2,800 BC) that mentions the applications of 366 plants. The Egyptian 'Ebers Papyrus' of 1500 BC gives us an insight into the use of medicinal plants during that period and region. The Egyptians used myrrh (*Commiphora molmol*), one of the three gifts of the Wise Men, as an incense to fumigate rooms and as a preservative in embalming. This tree is still widely used in herbal medicine today as a strong antiseptic. The Egyptians also had a sophisticated understanding of the medicinal value of scents, providing the early origins of aromatherapy.

A particularly significant text was the work of Pedanius Dioscorides, a Greek physician who served as a surgeon in the Roman army under the Emperor Nero. His masterwork of 78 AD is known by its Latin title, 'De Materia Medica', although its original Greek title translates as 'About Medicinal Trees'. This book contains references to 600 medicinal plants and was to remain highly influential for an astonishing 1,500 years. Galen (130–200 AD), who along with Hippocrates has had the most enduring impact on the practice of medicine, and who was a notoriously severe critic, said of Dioscorides 'In my opinion, he is among the authors who has presented the most perfect discussion of the drugs' – high praise indeed!

Many other texts have shaped the use and popularity of plant medicine over the centuries. Of particular note is John Gerard's 'Herbal or General Historie of Plantes' published in 1597, which was immensely popular. Even more successful was Nicholas Culpeper's 'Herbal' (originally titled 'The English Physician'). This is without doubt the most famous herbal we have; it was first published in 1652 and is still in print today!

Today we tend to overlook the fact that in the early twentieth century the practice of conventional medicine was still substantially founded on the use of plant medicines. I have a beautiful edition of 'The British Pharmaceutical Codex' of 1907 that is full of plant profiles. 'Southalls' Organic Materia Medica' written by John Barclay in 1909 for 'medical students, chemists, druggists and others' has a whole section devoted to 'barks' containing details of 40 tree barks then commonly in use in medicine. These included magnolia ('a mild stimulant, aromatic tonic and diaphoretic'), cinnamon ('as stomachic, carminative and mild astringent'), pomegranate ('as astringent and anthelmintic'), and Jamaica dogwood ('as sudorific, narcotic and anodyne' with a note that it 'has been employed for catching fish on account of its stupefying properties').

Two little-known herbal movements in America in the nineteenth and early twentieth centuries have had a profound effect on the professional practice of herbal medicine today. These were the Eclectics and the Physio-Medicalists. The leading light of the Eclectic movement was Dr Wooster Beach who, in his 'American Practice of Medicine' of 1831, rejected the use of blood-letting and poisonous medicines such as calomel, a compound containing mercury. Instead he called for an appreciation of the knowledge of indigenous 'root and Indian doctors' and extolled the virtues of plant remedies over mineral and synthetic medicines. The Eclectics benefited from having an exceptional pharmacist who specialized in developing high quality plant preparations; this was John Uri Lloyd of Lloyd Brothers Pharmacists. 'King's American Dispensatory' written by Dr John King and revised by Lloyd and another major Eclectic figure Dr Harvey W. Felter was published in 1897.

The Physio-Medicalists also reacted against the use of strong chemical remedies. In 'The Physio-Medical Dispensatory' (1869), one of the key writings produced by this approach, its author Dr William H. Cook explained that:

> The school of Physio-Medicalism… teaches that disease can be cured only by the use of such agencies as conform to the laws of Life and assist the powers of Nature. It rejects poisons of all kinds, and refuses a place in its Materia Medica to any article that tends to cause disease… It does not reject the old merely because it is old, nor accept the new merely because of its being new; but reads the open Book of Nature as the one grand source of earthly wisdom…

These two schools of thought deteriorated and slowly disappeared following an investigation into the state of medical schools conducted by the Carnegie Endowment for the Advancement of Teaching, following on from an initiative started by the Council on Medical Education of the American Medical Association. The investigation was led by Abraham Flexner and his report, delivered in 1910, pronounced that the standards of education in the Eclectic and Physio-Medical training colleges were poor. They never recovered from this indictment. Nonetheless many of their writings remain fascinating and relevant works, containing a wealth of knowledge about the applications of plant remedies.

One of the most important herbals of the twentieth century was 'The Modern Herbal' written by Maud Grieve (or Mrs M. Grieve, as the book cover had it), published in 1931. A Fellow of the Royal Horticultural Society she used her expertise during the Second World War, in response to demand for more medicines, to train people in the cultivation of healing plants. Her book is a huge compendium of medicinal plant profiles that had originally been written as individual pamphlets on each plant. Although no longer entirely 'modern' it is still a tremendously impressive and enjoyable work. It also stands as a landmark publication signalling the beginning of a resurgence of interest in herbal medicine.

TREE REMEDIES IN HISTORY

Cinchona

We can trace the development of the contemporary interest in trees from a scientific perspective back to the seventeenth century. Just 500 years ago the Old World and the New World had yet to come into contact with each other. This separation came to an end when the Spanish conquered the Inca Empire in Peru. One positive outcome of this invasion for the rest of the world, and certainly the most significant therapeutic export from South America to Europe, was the discovery of the use of Cinchona trees for the treatment of malaria. It may be forgotten now but at that time malaria was common in England and other European countries. It was the world's number one killer disease at the time.

Malaria is so-named because it was thought to be caused by bad ('mal') air emanating from swamps and marshy ground. In fact, it is due to infection with one of four species of a protozoan called *Plasmodium* that is transmitted by mosquito bites. It produces attacks of fever that occur at regular intervals (such as every other day or every three days) depending on the type of malaria. Cinchona was famous for the treatment of such periodic fevers in South America

Cinchona was introduced into Europe around 1630. Initially, it was known in Spain as 'quina-quina', meaning 'bark of barks' from which derives the name of the main active antimalarial constituent of Cinchona that was isolated in 1820 – quinine. Native South Americans knew it as 'fever tree', but it became most commonly known in the West as 'Peruvian bark', after its country of origin, or 'Jesuit's bark' because it was brought to the West by Jesuit missionaries.

The name Cinchona (which was not given to the tree until 1739) derives from what is now thought to be a myth about the discovery of this powerful medicine by the Spanish. The tale goes that the Countess of Cinchon, wife of the Viceroy of Peru, was cured of malaria by this tree and that afterwards her title was attached to it. The true story of how quinidine, another alkaloid constituent of Cinchona, was later discovered to be useful for heart irregularities is equally interesting. A Dutch patient consulted an eminent heart specialist in 1912 and told him that he had discovered a way to control his irregular pulse. He did it by taking one gram of quinine. In 1918 it was found that it was actually another alkaloid, quinidine, which was having the beneficial effect. Quinidine is still very important in the treatment of heart rhythm disturbances.

The demand for Cinchona bark soon became massive although it was slow to catch on in some quarters. It was introduced to England in the 1650s but was treated with suspicion by Protestants who saw it as a Catholic medicine. This wariness was so pronounced that Oliver Cromwell died of malaria in 1658 after having refused to be 'Jesuited' with Cinchona bark. It was also only slowly recommended by doctors who, perhaps, had been reluctant to diminish the trade in a disease they had hitherto found to be lucrative! Although quinine was identified as the main active constituent of Cinchona in 1820 it proved impossible to synthesize it, so the supply of quinine continued to rely on natural supplies of the bark. Demand was such that the bark became worth its weight in silver and the main Cinchona growing countries in South America (including Bolivia, Colombia and Ecuador, as well as Peru) tried to prevent the export of Cinchona seeds in order to preserve a monopoly on supply. Eventually, a Dutch botanist, Justus Hasskarl, succeeded in obtaining seeds and growing the trees in Java, Indonesia. Unfortunately for him the trees that eventually grew turned out to contain very little quinine.

There are at least 40 different species of Cinchona with the quinine content varying substantially between them – from high to very low. *Cinchona ledgeriana* is one of the higher-yielding species that was eventually identified by the Australian Charles Ledger, with the help of a Native Indian who was subsequently killed for this betrayal by the Bolivian government. The Dutch bought seeds from Ledger and developed extensive plantations in Java, subsequently gaining control of the quinine market. This proved to have dramatic consequences during the Second World War when a combination of the German occupation of Holland and the Japanese conquest of Indonesia took access to the world's major quinine stocks out of the hands of the Allies. Many Allied soldiers were at greater risk of death from malaria than from active combat and the lack of quinine became a serious problem.

A botanist, Raymond Fosberg, was appointed by the US government to travel to South America and identify and collect as great a quantity of Cinchona bark as was possible. Finding substantial colonies of the trees was not easy and it took Fosberg and his team months to locate supplies. During his work in South America, he was tracked down by two Nazi agents who cornered him in a hotel late one night. Fosberg feared for his life, but he was lucky – the agents revealed that they had been searching for him, not to kill him, but to offer a deal. They had defected and had a quantity of pure quinine, smuggled out of Germany, that they wished to sell to him. Fosberg struck the deal with huge relief.

Newer drugs have now largely superseded the role of quinine in the treatment of malaria, but we still use the synthetic chloroquine for malaria prevention. It is estimated that chloroquine is still the second most commonly used drug in the world (the number one spot is taken by another tree-derived drug – aspirin – of which more shortly).

Guaiac

Another tree from South America and the West Indies achieved great popularity in treating a severe and widespread disease in the sixteenth century, though its success was not to be as long-lived. The tree was *Guaiacum officinale* and the disease was syphilis. Again, the Spanish, this time in the Caribbean, observed the native use of Guaiacum, or guaiac as it was known, in treating the symptoms of syphilis. The 'cure' involved taking regular doses of guaiac, following strict dietary measures (including fasting) and being 'sweated' – enduring exposure to the hot sun or strongly heated rooms in order to raise the body temperature. The treatment lasted for around 40 days.

Guaiac was first brought across to Europe in 1508 from when it rapidly became much sought after by syphilitics. This is perhaps not surprising since their main other treatment option was to take highly toxic mercury compounds. Unfortunately, the craze for guaiac dwindled because it came to be seen as ineffective. This is probably because people were just taking the plant without following the original additional treatment strategies of diet and sweating, and not following the course for long enough.

Pau d'arco

Many medicines from the South American rain forest are still in use today. One of the most interesting is the tree known as pau d'arco (*Tabebuia* species) that has been used for over 1,000 years by Brazilian healers. These are beautiful tall trees with trumpet-like flowers.

In the 1960s the Brazilian media announced that a cure for cancer had at last been found – the bark of the pau d'arco tree. This statement was based on a series of anecdotal reports and the experiences of medical staff treating terminal cancer patients at a hospital in Sao Paulo, Brazil. Despite initial doubts, subsequent research has demonstrated that pau d'arco does indeed have some significant antitumour qualities. Certainly there is a strong traditional basis for its usefulness. The Mayan-speaking Haustec Indians have long used external applications of pau d'arco for wounds and have taken it by mouth for malaise and cancer. The Quollhuaya herbalists of the Bolivian Andes are respected as being the most knowledgeable traditional healers in the whole of South America and they also use pau d'arco for cancer and leukaemia.

Although it does have a role to play in aiding patients with cancer, the popularity of pau d'arco in the West today is based on its activity as an immune boosting herb. Extracts stimulate white blood cells (lymphocytes) that are involved in fighting disease. Pau d'arco is often helpful where there is a chronic lowered resistance to disease, for instance in individuals who seem constantly to contract coughs and colds. Research has shown it to be antifungal and it is used in treating infection with *Candida albicans* in conditions such as vaginal thrush and ringworm. Studies also suggest that it may be useful in controlling certain viral infections such as Epstein-Barr virus (EBV), the virus that causes glandular fever. EBV may also be the original trigger in some cases of chronic fatigue syndrome. This lends support to the use of pau d'arco in treating this common and controversial condition.

Nutmeg and Cloves

The Dutch established a base on Java in order to further the interests of the Dutch East India Company (VOC – Vereenigde Oost-Indische Compagnie) which was founded in 1602. The business interests of the VOC were focused on one commodity – spices. Of all the spices two trees mattered most – nutmeg (*Myristica fragrans*) and cloves (*Syzygium aromaticum*).

But the Dutch weren't the only nation interested in the spice trade, the English and Portuguese also wanted to control as much of the trade as they could. What we now term the spice trade might equally be called the spice wars. Conflict between the three European nations was severe and huge risks were taken to sail vast distances to Indonesia to recover the prized plants. Many sailors died during the long voyages and native islanders suffered terrible privations as battles were fought to control the Spice Islands.

Why were such exertions made, such dangers braved in order to secure a supply of spices that we now consider commonplace? Spices had always been highly prized for their culinary and medicinal virtues, as well as their rarity, but the price of nutmeg in particular rose beyond comprehension when Elizabethan physicians began to pronounce that it was the only sure cure for the plague. It was also very much in demand for its reputation as a potent aphrodisiac. It became worth more than its weight in gold and trading in it became a certain way of making a fortune. Its value is attested to by Samuel Pepys who, in 1665, recorded that he secretly handed over a sack full of gold to purchase a small pouch of nutmeg and cloves.

Nutmeg was one of the rarest of all spices, growing only on the six islands of Banda that cover just 40 square miles (104 square kilometres). They are now part of Indonesia, which was then called the East Indies. The Portuguese had been the first Western nation to land there in 1512. For centuries before then, spices had been traded through Venice. The spice route to Venice was complex, with native traders in Indonesia supplying fellow traders from India who in turn negotiated with Arabian merchants who brought the spices to Egypt. Constantinople was the main spice source for the Venetians.

The Arabians kept details of the origins of the spices a close secret and the Venetians did not know where their treasures actually came from. The Portuguese gradually penetrated the veil of mystery, beginning with Vasco da Gama's voyage to India in 1498 and culminating in the landing at the Banda islands. Portuguese dominance shifted the centre of the spice trade from Venice to Lisbon. But with the inflated plague prices, the Dutch and English wanted to cut out the middlemen and set out to capture as much of the market as they could, at source.

Today nutmeg and cloves are grown widely throughout tropical Asia to Australia. Though not as highly prized as before they remain valuable medicines and culinary items. Cloves particularly continue to be important for treating infections, pain and digestive disorders.

Aspirin

In the eighteenth century quinine was still very popular and was used to treat fevers of all kinds, not just malaria. But it was very expensive and this moved people to try and find substitutes for it. The Reverend Edward Stone noticed, in 1763, that powdered willow bark tasted somewhat similar to quinine and he tried it as a replacement for the South American drug in fevers, with good results. It was not until 1830 that the active constituent, salicin, was identified.

In 1835 salicylic acid was developed from salicylaldehyde extracted not from willow but from the herb meadowsweet (originally called *Spiraea ulmaria* but now renamed *Filipendula ulmaria*). In 1874 salicylic acid was produced synthetically. But it was not until 1899 that aspirin (acetylsalicylic acid) was first marketed by the Bayer Pharmaceutical Company. The name aspirin comes from Spiraea in acknowledgement of meadowsweet but 'salicylic' refers to the compound found in willows and called after their botanical name of *Salix*.

Aspirin became the most commonly used drug in the world, being used for fevers, headaches, arthritis and period pains amongst other complaints. It does, however, have one serious side effect – it can cause bleeding from the stomach. For this reason it is often substituted these days by other medications that are classed as non-steroidal anti-inflammatory drugs (NSAIDs) such as ibuprofen. An important new role has since been developed for aspirin by making a virtue out of the mechanism that causes its side effect. It is a reliable anticoagulant and is taken by millions of at risk people every day to thin the blood and help to prevent strokes and heart attacks. Though willow bark does not contain aspirin itself (it contains salicin which the body converts to salicylic acid), it is still a good treatment for fevers and arthritis, and it does not cause bleeding. It is still widely used by herbalists today.

MODERN RESEARCH

Around 25% of all prescription drugs are still derived from plants. Clues for the development of new conventional medicines are constantly being found in trees. Some current examples include:

- yew trees (*Taxus* species) and hazels (*Corylus avellana*) yield taxol which is used in the treatment of ovarian and breast cancer;

- *Maytenus* species, a group of African and South American trees, produce a chemical called maytansine that shows promise for leukaemia;

- Camptothecins from the Chinese tree *Camptotheca acuminata* are of value for lymphoma and hepatoma (a tumour of the liver);

- betulinic acid from the bark of the white birch (*Betula alba*) is being investigated as a treatment for skin cancer;

- the twigs and leaves of *Calophyllum lanigerum* yield calanolide A which has shown effectiveness in the test tube against the Human Immuno-deficiency Virus (HIV) that is associated with the development of AIDS;

- the Samoan mamala tree (*Homalanthus nutans*) contains a compound called prostratin which has also demonstrated promise in treating HIV infection.

The contribution of trees to medicine continues to evolve. While conventional medicine continues to source new drugs from plants, the traditional use of plants in herbal medicine and other complementary therapies is showing signs of vigorous health. In China herbal medicine is fully integrated into the mainstream health care system. Doctors in hospitals and surgeries prescribe herbal medicine alongside conventional drugs. In Germany and, to a lesser extent, France, herbal medicines are routinely prescribed by doctors. One of the most commonly prescribed of all drugs available to the modern general practitioner in these countries is *Ginkgo biloba*, which is given for a variety of circulatory problems.

There is substantial specialist training available to practitioners of traditional Chinese medicine in China and of Ayurvedic medicine in India, but in the West herbs are usually obtained over-the-counter from health food shops, and pharmacies, and occasionally from doctors. Throughout the West there is a lack of dedicated full professional training in herbal medicine. The exception to this is in the UK where The National Institute of Medical Herbalists was founded in 1864 as the professional body for medical herbalists – it has provided a specialized training in this discipline ever since.

The best way we have of assessing the present popularity of herbal remedies is by looking at sales figures. These are often difficult to quantify exactly but estimates have been made:

- total annual sales of herbal medicines across Europe in 1991 were £1.45 billion;

- total annual sales of herbal medicines in the UK was valued at £38 million, but this is likely to be a large underestimate as top-selling products such as ginkgo and garlic were excluded from the survey;

- total annual sales of herbal medicines in Germany in 1997 were US$1.8 billion;

- total annual sales of herbal medicines in France in 1997 were US$1.1 billion;

- in the USA, total annual herbal sales rose from US$1.6 billion in 1994 to US$4 billion in 1998.

Clearly, the demand for plant medicines is strong. Tree medicines continue to emerge to meet the need for safe and effective natural remedies.

3

The Forest Pharmacy – How Tree Medicines Work

TREE MEDICINES work in a number of radically different ways. Their effects can be divided into four broad categories.

Pharmacological

The mechanisms by which tree-based remedies work in medical systems such as herbal and conventional medicine are generally well recognized. The chemicals in trees are used by these systems to have direct effects on the body's physiological functioning. This way of working with trees can be described as pharmacologically based.

Ethereal (or Energetic)

In therapies such as homeopathy and flower remedies the mode of action is less clear. Such remedies use trees as a starting point for making medicines but they are prepared in a very dilute way – generally with no discernible trace of actual tree chemicals within them. This is not to say that such remedies do not work. While there has been very little research into flower remedies, there have been some studies that suggest the effectiveness of homeopathy, particularly in the treatment of animals.

A way has not yet been found to understand how these approaches work on a scientific level and further studies are needed. These types of medicines are often classed as being 'energetic', meaning they work with some kind of subtle energy, beyond the more physical chemical-based pharmacological approach. To label these systems as 'energetic' might be misleading since all therapeutic interventions can be described as working by means of energetic processes. Perhaps it is better to class them as 'ethereal' to imply that they may work by acting on more subtle channels of influence as yet poorly understood.

Psychological

Yet another group of therapies using trees as healing agents can be classed as psychological approaches. These include art therapy and meditation. Often the word 'psychological' is used dismissively, and is associated with the phrase 'it's all in the mind'. This belittling of a hugely important part of our health and well-being stems from the classical dissociation of links between mind and body. But it is inaccurate and harmful to view these two as being separate – we all have physical and psychological needs and activities. A particular illness can be principally focused as either physical or psychological but there is always a corresponding influence in the other. For example, a minor physical illness such as acne may lower a person's self-confidence causing them to become withdrawn and depressed. Similarly, the psychological condition of depression can lead to physical experiences of fatigue and debility. It is important that we work on both levels when treating any health disorder. The psychological methods of working with trees can have profound healing effects.

Physical

In addition, it is possible to describe the use of lubricating tree oils in the many forms of massage as having a physical effect on the body.

The use of tree medicines used in therapies in these four categories is summarized in the box on page 38.

There is an overlap between many of these categories and you will learn more about this as we look at each approach in turn. It is enough to say that it is rare for a medicine to only act on one level. Even when we take a conventional drug, the way we feel about that drug will influence how it acts upon us. If we welcome the treatment and feel positive about it then it is more likely to suit us and be more effective. Conversely, if we resent the drug and feel anxious about it then we may be more likely to experience side effects from taking it.

Pharmacological
Herbal medicine
Conventional drugs
Aromatic medicine
Aromatherapy
Nutritional medicine

Ethereal
Homeopathy
Flower remedies

Psychological
Art therapy
Stress therapy
Meditation

Physical
Massage
Touch therapy

It is tempting to try and link the categories of therapeutic approach with the definition of the levels upon which the body works – physical, emotional, mental and spiritual – but there is no close fit as several therapies can work on more than one level. For example, massage may appear to be a purely physical activity, working on relaxing muscles, but it can also produce feelings of great emotional and mental well-being. In people who have been sexually abused or who have issues about being physically touched, massage can trigger profound emotional release and healing. In the same way, it can be argued that while the 'ethereal' therapies may work on higher subtle spiritual energies homeopathy is also considered to be capable of producing marked physical reactions.

Today, the theoretical basis of medicine is starting to move away from the outdated mind–body dichotomy towards an integrated view of how we function. This is perhaps best demonstrated in an emerging scientific approach to the body with a very long name – psychoneuroendocrinoimmunology! This is often slightly shortened to psychoneuroimmunology or PNI. In the long version we can break down the meaning of the word as follows:

Psycho – the influence of the mind;

Neuro – the nervous system that carries signals to and from the mind;

Endocrino – the endocrine or hormonal system of the body;

Immunology – the way our bodies resist infectious and other disease.

If we put the whole word back together again, then in essence what it means is that this approach recognizes that there is a connection between what we think and how the body functions.

PNI stresses that what we think mentally and how we react emotionally will influence how we feel physically, and vice versa. It has been discovered, for instance, that laughter and its accompanying sensation of well-being can cause a rise in the white blood cells in our immune system that are responsible for fighting disease. There is a strong connection between our mental and emotional states and the major control systems of our bodies – the hormonal and immune systems. PNI helps explain how psychological methods such as meditation can cause positive changes in our physical health.

True health is not merely the absence of disease but is a multi-dimensional experience of physical, emotional, mental and spiritual well-being. Below you will discover the mechanism behind how each therapy works, the final section being an in-depth look at herbal medicine.

Massage

Massage works primarily by the application of pressure delivered by the hands (and sometimes elbows and feet) to the person being treated. Movement of the muscles and surrounding tissues increases circulation to the skin, muscles and internal organs improving their circulation, nutrition, oxygenation and relaxation. This can release tension, relieve pain and stiffness and promote better general bodily function.

The role of tree medicines here is primarily to provide lubricating fixed oils (*see* Herbal Medicine below) that give a medium for the massage practitioner to help work the muscles without making the skin dry or sore. But there is more to it than that. Certain oils have particular properties that can enhance the effectiveness of the massage treatment. Avocado oil is rich in vitamins A, D and E and can help to regenerate devitalized and aged skin. Hazelnut oil is slightly drying and can be used to improve oily skin. Peach kernel oil has a good vitamin A content and macadamia nut oil is also highly nutritive and restorative to sun-damaged and aged skin. Walnut oil contains gamma-linoleic acid (GLA) that has anti-inflammatory properties and can be used on sensitive and allergic skin.

Massage is one of the prime methods that aromatherapists use in applying volatile (essential) oils to the body.

Nutritional medicine

Nutritionists use tree products to improve dietary intake of valuable nutrients. This includes the use of tree fruits and nuts to help promote optimal nutrition. The body cannot function properly without an adequate nutritional intake. Tree medicines work in facilitating good health by providing substances that treat nutritional imbalances (either deficiencies or excesses – such as cholesterol) and by enhancing the body's health promoting functions (such as vitamin C stimulating the immune system).

The obvious nutritive content of nuts and fruits, such as vitamins, minerals, essential fatty acids, sugars and proteins, is supplemented by other plant chemicals. These include trace elements (for example, chromium, obtained from nuts, which is important to aid sugar metabolism – deficiency of chromium is associated with anxiety and fatigue) and antioxidants. Anthocyanins are potent antioxidants that provide the red, violet and blue colours in fruits such as cherries, plums and olives. They reduce free radical damage to the body's cells. This has the result of strengthening the circulation, helping to prevent the adverse effects of ageing, reducing the risk of cancer and decreasing the risk and symptoms of inflammatory disorders such as arthritis.

Conventional medicine

Orthodox medicine uses drugs derived from trees to treat various conditions. Usually, the aim is to isolate the most useful active chemical from a particular therapeutic tree and then reproduce it synthetically in the laboratory and give it to patients in a purified and standardized form.

Such tree-based drugs work in the same way as any other conventional drug – by having a direct chemical effect on the body's internal functioning. Such treatments can be potent and fast acting but carry higher risks of causing side effects than the other tree medicine systems.

Aromatic medicine and aromatherapy

Both aromatic medicine and aromatherapy use volatile oils (*see* Herbal Medicine below) to promote health and treat disease. Aromatic medicine is distinguished from aromatherapy in that it uses volatile oils both internally and externally on the body whereas aromatherapy focuses on external application and does not give volatile oils by mouth.

Volatile (essential) oils have marked pharmacological properties. Almost all volatile oils are markedly antimicrobial, acting against bacteria (such as tea tree, *Melaleuca alternifolia*), fungi (for example, tree of life, *Thuja occidentalis*) and even viruses (including *Ravensara aromatica* – a Madagascan tree). These oils can also relieve pain, relax muscular spasms and stimulate the circulation. Some volatile oils can be taken by mouth following expert professional advice but are usually applied by massaging on the skin or by inhalation. Inhalations can deliver the antiseptic oil molecules into the nose and airways thereby having direct effects on infections in the sinuses and lungs. Consequently, volatile oils have a strong reputation for treating respiratory tract infections.

Aromatherapy also claims to be able to influence our emotional and mental health. Inhalation of volatile oils introduces their effects into the brain by way of stimulation of the olfactory nerves. Studies have shown that different scents have differently shaped molecules that fit an array of 'smell receptors' in the olfactory system. The olfactory nerves connect with a part of the brain called the limbic system; this is commonly described as 'the seat of the emotions'. This area is associated with memory and with emotional and sexual responses and the feeling of hunger.

Most of us have noticed that a particular smell can trigger off certain memories or emotions, and that some smells are evocative – the scent of wood smoke on crisp autumn days, the chill night air in winter, spicy cinnamon creating a sense of Christmas, or a particular smell associated with childhood. As for sexual stimulation, this has kept the perfume industry in business for hundreds of years! Looked at in this way it is easy to appreciate why the inhalation of volatile oils influences our mood, appetite and libido.

Art therapy

Art therapy uses a number of strategies to achieve improvements in physical and mental health. Trees can be used as a focus for various art media such as drawing, painting, poetry and photography.

The power of trees to inspire is attested to by the painter Harold Hitchcock, a descendant of the famous artist George Stubbs. As his biographer Emmanuel Williams has described, Hitchcock had a visionary experience with trees as a boy. Walking out early one morning he witnessed a glorious sunrise that emerged from behind a stand of old elm trees. He was moved by the interplay of light and leaves and this vision so affected him that it formed the foundation of his life's work. I think the way Hitchcock describes his experience says a lot about the way that nature can awaken and motivate us:

> It was that one moment that touched something off in me, and made me wish to recapture it through painting. There was a wonderful feeling of harmony and well-being and peace. In particular the sunlight on the

bark and roots of the trees presented a scintillating, jewel-like vision of colour. I remember saying to myself that I would not rest until I had somehow recaptured something of this vision or experience.

Williams attests to the power of Hitchcock's art by observing that it 'takes us into the primeval garden, into a state – rather than a location – that feels like Eden. There is no greater gift than this.'

We cannot all have the skill of a painter like Hitchcock in being able to translate what we feel so powerfully. But we can all share a visionary experience and discover more about ourselves and our world by trying to investigate and interpret this experience artistically.

Creativity is the key to positive change and it can be triggered by encounters with trees and then channelled through art therapy. This process can be helpful in conditions such as depression and also when recovering from severe illness. It works by accessing the beauty and wonder that trees can generate and by providing a way in which we can instil such life enhancing feelings within ourselves. The result can be to give us hope and comfort, and engender a sense of meaning and purpose. By feeling a connection with nature we are spurred to recovery. Such positive feelings imbue the body with a spiritual sustenance that supports the healing process.

Stress therapy

The treatment of stress can take many forms depending on the cause of the stress and the circumstances and personality of the person experiencing it. Spending time with trees, just being in their presence, can be of benefit in easing the common stresses of a busy life.

One of the most significant stressors in modern times is the sheer speed with which we live our lives. We travel rapidly and frequently by car, air travel opens up the whole world to us almost at an instant, and computers and the Internet respond to our requests almost quicker than we can formulate our thoughts. Long hours of intellectual work and the growing problem of information overload stress our minds. We often have too much to do and not enough time to do it in.

Family life and work patterns are changing significantly and while this may bring benefits it also presents us with challenges. Constant developments in technology are forever creating new issues and concerns (such as genetic modification of foods). We can worry about HIV, BSE, the state of the environment and what kind of world we will leave to our children and grandchildren... Sometimes it can all become just too much.

The value of trees is that we can go to them and draw on their stillness, their emanations of permanence and peace. Sometimes when we are with trees, especially in their natural habitats in the wild, we can feel their 'wisdom'. Trees do not run about all over the place, they develop slowly and they follow regular patterns and cycles. They are beautiful, natural and graceful. Older trees often have an impressive quality that I can only describe as dignity.

To be with healthy undamaged trees is to draw upon a deep well of strength and peace. Different species have different characters that are not necessarily universal; characters that we all interpret differently. For me, mature beech trees have an aura of grandeur and majesty, they are like monarchs or emperors and to be in their presence in beech woods is like visiting a castle or a great cathedral. The experience is elevating and profound. A field of low coppiced willows and osiers of many shades of green, red and gold, being cultivated for basket making, has a different character again. Such a collection of colourful and carefully husbanded trees is scintillating, harmonious and joyous.

Trees work to relieve stress by slowing us down, reconnecting us to the earth, giving us back a sense of belonging, instilling beauty in our hearts and peace in our minds. All it takes is to seek trees out and simply be with them. The roots of trees knit the earth together and they can also hold us together at the times when we are finding it difficult to cope.

Meditation and visualization

While going out to spend time with trees in gardens or in the wild can be wonderfully healing there are many times when this may not be possible. At such times we can find a space to be where we can visualize a particular tree, forest, tree symbol or image and meditate on its meaning. This practice can bring all the benefits of stress therapy. We can also use meditation while sitting with trees outdoors; this can bring about a feeling of closer kinship with the tree and provide a starting point from which to 'leap off' to explore other feelings and ideas.

Studies have shown that visualization techniques and meditation can lower blood pressure and raise white blood cell counts in the immune system. Spiritual healers use these strategies to imagine their patients becoming well. Scientific research has demonstrated that our physiological functioning changes during meditation. Further research could tell us a lot more about the healing power of the mind and show us new ways in which we can work with the concept of PNI to prevent and treat disease. For many healthcare practitioners this, rather than gene therapy, represents the future of medicine.

The explanation given by esoteric writers as to how meditation and visualization work is that 'energy follows thought'. This means that if we create a 'thought form' by means of focused and consistent use of the mind it will eventually become embodied in reality. The theory is that by working with images of trees and thinking ourselves into the trees' spirit we can access the healing powers of trees at a mental or spiritual level.

Homeopathy

Homeopathy uses plants and other substances to create medicinal remedies. A number of trees, such as thuja (*Thuja occidentalis*), are used. The concept behind homeopathy is that of 'like cures like'. Some substances, including certain trees, can cause symptoms (usually only when taken in excess, at the level of an 'overdose') that are similar to certain disease states. Homeopaths believe that when the symptoms of a particular disease state match the symptom picture of a certain substance then if you give a very small amount of that substance it will cure the disease. Hence 'like cures like'.

When I said a 'very small' amount, I meant very, very small! Most homeopathic preparations are so dilute that it is impossible to detect any of the original substance's chemicals in the preparation. Not only this, homeopaths contend that the weaker the concentration of the original therapeutic substance – the *stronger* will be the effect on the body. The obvious problem for conventional scientists is that this concept flies in the face of the known laws of physics and biochemistry!

Whether homeopathy really does have beneficial effects and how these effects are caused are questions to which we still have no conclusive answers. One theory is that the way that homeopathic remedies are prepared, by repeatedly diluting them and shaking ('succussing') them in water somehow interacts with water molecules suffusing them with the essence of the substance being extracted. It is possible that science will one day make new discoveries that will explain how homeopathy works, but for now it remains a mystery. The main evidence we have to show that this treatment works are the clinical experiences of many homeopaths and their patients.

Flower remedies

Flower remedies are made from all kinds of flowering plants including trees. They are prepared in a similar way to homeopathic remedies and the same issues about whether and how they work apply. However, unlike homeopathic medicines, they are prescribed to treat psychological rather than physical symptoms.

Though many complementary medicine practitioners prescribe flower remedies, they are most often self-prescribed. It is possible to buy books listing the psychological states that flower remedies can treat, decide which state most closely matches one's own and then take the appropriate flower remedy. It is not to belittle the potential value of flower remedies to say that there is probably a large placebo effect to be derived from using psychological state descriptions to think about where our problems lie and upon which levels we therefore need to work. It is possible that at least some of the effects that flower remedies produce can be attributed to this.

A special photographic technique called Kirlian photography has been used to take pictures of 'energetic medicines' such as flower remedies. These photographs appear to show a vibrant aura of light emanating from flower remedies. The qualities that flower remedies capture from trees and other plants are thought to be their more subtle energies that exert an influence at higher mental and spiritual levels. By contrast herbal remedies are thought, according to this view, to capture the more physical and tangible characteristics of tree medicines.

Herbal medicine

In ancient times people used herbs because they had observed that they worked. The issue of *how* they worked exactly was not of primary importance, although people have always sought to understand the processes involved.

In traditional Chinese medicine, herbs are still understood to work according to principles first established several thousands of years ago. A Chinese herbalist will talk about herbs working by 'moving the spleen' or clearing 'blood stagnation'. Greek and Arabian medical writings of the Middle Ages, which came to predominate in the West and which form the origins of our modern medicine, speak of herbs working by influencing the 'four humours'. These are yellow bile, black bile, blood and phlegm. Herbs were classified with reference to their physical characteristics (or 'qualities') according to temperature and moisture in varying degrees, for example, chilli peppers (*Capsicum minimum*) would be classed as 'hot and dry in the first degree'.

Such understanding of how herbs work was based on close study of plants and by observation on their interactions with people. A new interpretation of herbal activity came about following the invention of the microscope and the development of new techniques in chemical analysis.

The unravelling of the chemical structure of herbs progressed alongside new findings about their functioning. By linking the chemistry of plants with the chemistry of the body it became possible to see how herbal medicines act to improve human health. However, some discoveries merely gave new names and finer detail to effects that had been well-known by traditional healers for many generations. Volatile oils (*see* below) had been distilled from aromatic plants by the Egyptians who used them for their antiseptic qualities without being aware of the existence of the infectious micro-organisms that the oils were killing off. By the time they were named, the constituents known as tannins (*see* below) had long been used for their secretion-binding and tissue-tightening effects in treating diarrhoea and other disorders. All the same, chemical discoveries have led to a great leap forward in our knowledge of how plants work.

It could be argued that, if we can see that plant medicines *do* work, do we really need to know *how* they work? The answer is 'yes,' for several reasons. By knowing how a plant achieves its effects we can be more accurate in prescribing it – using it only when we know it is likely to help, avoiding its use in people who might be adversely affected by it, and giving it at the right dose and in the best type of preparation. When exploring the chemistry and activity of plants we can also discover new things about them. For example research into *Ginkgo biloba* found that it had a hitherto unknown action in decreasing certain allergic responses. As a consequence of this discovery I now routinely use ginkgo leaves in the treatment of asthma, with good results. By knowing how herbs work we can use them with greater confidence in their safety and efficacy.

Over the last few decades, herbal remedies have been researched more and more extensively. Herbal medicine is today the most heavily researched of all the complementary therapies. Not all of this research is of equal value. Some research is more useful than others – for instance, looking at isolated single chemicals from plants and testing them 'in vitro' (meaning outside of the body, or 'in the test tube') is of less significance than exploring the use of whole herb preparations 'in vivo' (meaning taken inside the body). While many high-quality human clinical trials have been carried out, there remains very little research data about many medicinal trees and there remains an urgent need for more studies to be conducted.

A proper understanding of how herbs work is achieved by carefully comparing the insights of science with the body of traditional wisdom that has built up around a particular plant. Having said this, it is extremely useful to understand the specific types of chemicals that healing plants contain. It needs to be borne in mind that we never give just one type of chemical in herbal practice. Each particular plant represents a mix of hundreds of different chemicals although often one particular active group may predominate. Also, herbalists usually prescribe more than one plant at a time, thereby increasing the chemical complexity of the medicine. An important concept in herbalism is that of synergy – meaning that therapeutic plants (and the chemicals they are made of) work better when skilfully combined and prescribed together.

Before exploring the active chemical constituents of medicinal trees in detail it is useful to reflect on why trees produce such substances. Most of the chemicals listed below are described as 'secondary metabolites'.

Primary metabolites are substances known to be essential to the development of plants, such as sugars, acids, proteins and fats. Many primary metabolites are central to the value of tree products used in nutritional medicine.

Secondary metabolites, on the other hand, were once considered to represent the plants' waste products. We now know that many of these substances are of vital importance to the survival of plants. A great number of them are involved in defence and repair strategies. Alkaloids, for instance, can poison herbivorous animals thus deterring them from eating the plants. Resins are secreted when trees are physically damaged, helping to seal the wound and destroy any infection that might develop. Tannins prevent wood from decaying as a result of microbial and insect attacks. Coumarins prevent germination of seeds until the time is right for this to happen. If the seed germinates too soon it may not survive. Secondary metabolites demonstrate the intimate and harmonious relationship we have with the plant kingdom.

ACTIVE CHEMICAL CONSTITUENTS OF MEDICINAL TREES

Alkaloids

These are nitrogen-containing plant products that are often highly toxic but can have very rapid and powerful healing effects. Tree medicines possessing them are of value in treating severe or emergency conditions. Such trees need to be treated with great caution and should only usually be taken following expert professional advice. An example is the poison nut tree (*Strychnos nux-vomica*) which contains the alkaloid strychnine. There are several categories of alkaloids such as indole alkaloids, pyrrolizidine alkaloids and tropane alkaloids.

Alkaloids can have several beneficial properties, including relieving pain, lowering blood pressure, opening up the airways (bronchodilator), and treating infections and cancers. Boldine, an alkaloid from the Chilean boldo tree (*Peumus boldo*), stimulates the gall bladder and is useful for gallstones. The Australian corkwood trees (*Duboisia myoporoides* and *Duboisia leichhardtii*) contain high concentrations of atropine and are used in place of the original herbaceous source of atropine (deadly nightshade, *Atropa belladonna*) to provide commercial supplies of this important drug.

Coumarins

Coumarins smell of new mown hay and have several actions including antifungal and anticoagulant – the conventional blood-thinning drug warfarin is a synthetic derivative of plant coumarins. Furanocoumarins are use to treat vitiligo and psoriasis in conjunction with UV light exposure. Trees containing coumarins include citrus trees and the fig tree (*Ficus carica*).

Fixed oils

Fixed oils are distinguished from volatile oils. When poured onto a surface, volatile oils, as the name suggests, evaporate away leaving hardly any trace of themselves but fixed oils remain as a greasy pool. You will know fixed oils better as vegetable oils and they include familiar cooking oils such as olive oil. They are mostly obtained by pressing tree fruits. Other fixed tree oils include apricot kernel, avocado, hazelnut, macadamia nut, sweet almond and walnut oils. All of these are used as massage oils to improve skin tone.

Flavonoids

This group of chemicals includes flavones, flavonols and anthocyanins. They usually occur attached to sugars as glycosides (*see* below). They tend to be yellow pigments ('flavonoids' derives from flavus, the Latin for yellow). Anthocyanins give the red, violet and blue-black colours to flowers and fruits. Once viewed as waste products, it now appears that they play several important roles including regulating plant growth, protecting plants from harmful UV radiation and providing defence against infection. In humans they stabilize the bodies membranes and are strong antioxidants. They help to improve the condition of the heart and circulation and protect us against the effects of environmental stress.

Glycosides

A glycoside is any plant chemical that has a sugar attached to it. When we swallow them they are broken down to separate the sugar from the more active plant chemical (known as the 'aglycone') which then goes on to exert its effects.

There are a large number of different plant glycosides including the flavonoids (*see* above) and saponins (*see* below). Cyanogenic glycosides release hydrogen cyanide when they are broken down, and they are present in several members of the cherry family (*Rosaceae*); wild cherry (*Prunus serotina*) is used to treat coughs largely because of its cyanogenic glycoside content. Antraquinones are glycosides that are strong laxatives, they occur in trees such as cascara sagrada (*Rhamnus purshiana*) and should be avoided during pregnancy as they can have a stimulant effect on the pregnant uterus.

Gums

Gums are polysaccharides (sugar complexes) that form sticky masses. They are produced by plants to plug wounds, sealing them off from infection. Tree gums include gum arabic (*Acacia senegal*).

Mucilages

Like gums, mucilages are also polysaccharides. They are plant substances that readily absorb water and swell to make a slimy gel. In plants they are mainly concerned with retaining water – for instance, they often coat seeds, thus providing a means of keeping water at close hand for use during germination.

One of the most noted tree mucilages is the powdered inner bark of slippery elm (*Ulmus rubra*). Mucilage preparations have a soothing effect on the body's internal lining (mucous membranes) and externally on the skin. Mucilaginous pastes are wonderful for coating inflamed and sore areas of the digestive system in conditions such as heartburn (reflux oesophagitis) and colitis.

Napthoquinones

These are quinone-based chemicals that can be antibacterial and antifungal. They include juglone from the leaves of the walnut (*Juglans regia*) and butternut (*Juglans cinerea*) and lapachol from pau d'arco (*Tabebuia* species).

Resins

Resins are mixtures of chemicals, mainly acids, esters and terpenoids, which are secreted when trees are wounded. They do not dissolve in water but will readily mix with alcohol. Because of this they are usually prescribed as tinctures (water/alcohol liquid herbal preparations). They are common in conifers such as pine trees and the New Zealand kauri tree (*Agathis australis*).

Frankincense (*Boswellia sacra*) and myrrh (*Commiphora molmol*) are both resins; in common with most resins this famous pair are aromatic (the resin contains a volatile oil). Resins are highly antimicrobial, for example, the resinous compound called mastic (mastic tree, *Pistacia lentiscus*) is effective against the bacterium that causes stomach ulcers (*Helicobacter pylori*).

Saponins

Saponins derive their name from their tendency to produce a foam when shaken. They are bitter tasting, can be toxic to animals, and have been used as fish poisons (for example Jamaica dogwood, *Piscidia erythrina*). It is thought that saponins help plants to deter predators. As medicines they have a number of uses such as improving the integrity of the walls of veins (horse chestnut, *Aesculus hippocastanum*) making them useful in treating varicose veins and haemorrhoids, and lowering blood cholesterol levels – the saponins in limeflowers (*Tilia* species) have this effect.

Tannins

Tannins bind proteins and pull animal membranes tightly together, acting as an astringent agent. The puckering effect of drinking a really strong cup of China tea on the skin lining the mouth is an astringent effect caused by the presence of tannins. Tannins (traditionally derived from oak galls) are used to 'tan' animal hides, converting them to leather. Tannins are present in all tree barks.

Notable sources of medicinal tannins include oak bark (*Quercus robur*) and witch hazel bark and leaves (*Hamamelis virginiana*). Tannins bind secretions and are of great value in treating diarrhoea, dysentery and wounds. They staunch bleeding and bind skin proteins together creating a leathery scar very quickly. They are also useful for heavy menstrual bleeding and in reducing inflammatory swellings and can be antibacterial and antiviral.

Tannins are divided into two groups – hydrolysable (dissolving easily in water) and condensed (only partially soluble in water and alcohol). Condensed tannins can be excellent antioxidants, offering profound health benefits due to their effects in reducing cellular damage. Both green tea and red wine are good sources of beneficial condensed tannins. A class of condensed tannins called oligomeric procyanidins (OPCs), or pycnogenols, possess potent antioxidant activity helping to promote a healthy vascular system. OPCs are present in pine bark and hawthorn trees (*Crataegus* species).

The drawback with tannins is that they can bind with nutrients in the diet, or other herbs in a prescription, thus reducing their availability to the body. It is certainly not a good idea to drink too much strong China tea as this can lead to nutritional depletion.

Volatile oils

Volatile (essential) oils are very complex aromatic compounds. They are responsible for the scents of trees such as pine, cinnamon and clove. They are usually extracted by means of steam distillation and the vast majority are colourless.

Pure distilled volatile oils are used in aromatic medicine and aromatherapy but in herbal medicine they are usually left within the original plant part that contains them – such as leaf or flower. They contain many different chemicals (often over 50) including monoterpenes (an example of which is cineole found in many trees including *Eucalyptus* species), sesquiterpenes, alcohols, aldehydes, ketones (such as thujone from the tree of life, *Thuja occidentalis*), phenols (such as eugenol from cloves, *Syzygium aromaticum*), esters, ethers and oxides. Volatile oils can have many actions including antimicrobial, relaxant, circulatory stimulation and immune boosting.

4

Spreading Branches –
The Main Strands of Tree
Medicine

NOW WE HAVE looked at the ways in which tree medicines are thought to work, it is time to see how they can be used in practice. We will look at the methods or preparations peculiar to each therapy and how these can be applied to enhance our general sense of well-being or to treat particular conditions.

Some medicines and treatments that are for professional use only are also mentioned. In such cases the need for professional advice is pointed out. However, we will focus on the things that you can do for yourself at home, helping you create a state of optimal health, and also for the treatment of the minor problems of everyday life.

This is a mainly hands-on chapter dealing with the practical uses of trees, so before going any further it will be useful to remember a few points about tree medicine safety. Some of the therapies don't involve using tree products in a physical way at all. A practice such as meditation clearly carries few safety issues. Flower remedies contain no detectable tree chemicals and so they also can be considered very safe. It is important not to rely on flower remedies alone if you have a moderate to severe medical condition or if your problem is failing to clear up or is becoming worse. As for other tree medicines taken by mouth there is a general rule that the more chemically complex the medicine is the safer it is likely to be. Tree foods and herbal medicines are complex mixes of hundreds of tree chemicals and can broadly (though not always) be considered safer than semi-complex tree preparations (volatile oils) and simple tree remedies (conventional drugs).

When making up tree medicines, remember good basic hygiene such as washing your hands before and after making a preparation. With volatile oils it is particularly important to wash your hands after handling them because otherwise you may touch your eyes or other sensitive areas with traces of these strong substances and this can cause considerable stinging pain and discomfort.

Aromatic Medicine and Aromatherapy

What are they?

These systems of healing are based on the therapeutic qualities of volatile (essential) oils. Volatile oils are aromatic plant constituents that can be obtained from raw plant materials by distillation. Volatile oils are generally, but not always, pleasant smelling and nearly all of them have strong anti-septic qualities. Many plant parts yield volatile oils including barks, leaves, flowers, fruit rinds and seeds. The oils are frequently very strong when purified from the original plant matter and need to be handled with care. They are often corrosive when neat and need to be diluted before using. You should always wash your hands immediately after handling these oils to avoid rubbing them into sensitive areas such as the eyes.

The practice of using purified volatile oils as medicines goes back at least to Egyptian times but their use was not embodied in any particular approach with its own philosophy of practice. Rather, volatile oils were seen as being merely one therapeutic substance amongst others of vegetable, animal or mineral origin and were used as one element in the pharmacy of general medicine. Many herbalists today feel that the use of volatile oils belongs properly within the practice of herbal medicine since all volatile oils derive from plants. Having said this, there is a view among some of the more traditional herbalists that only whole plant medicines can constitute herbal remedies and that 'semi-purified' plant products such as volatile oils should be dealt with by a separate medical system

The discipline of aromatherapy has evolved, most extensively in the UK, centred on the use of volatile oils. This consists of conventional massage techniques but with the addition of volatile oils to the standard fixed carrier oils used in traditional massage. Other methods of application of volatile oils used by aromatherapists include baths, steam inhalations and the diffusion of scents within rooms. Aromatherapy tends to retain a focus on treating psychological states and has attained a reputation for treating conditions of tension and stress. As such it has become perceived as a 'relaxation therapy'. The tendency for many aromatherapists to practice from 'beauty parlours' rather than clinics and the oft repeated encouragement to 'pamper yourself with essential oils' has undermined the serious medical benefits that volatile oils can offer. This has resulted in a popular perception of aromatherapy as simply 'fragrant massage'.

The concept of aromatic medicine developed in France to promote the advantages that volatile oils can offer in treating physical disorders. In addition to the application routes used by aromatherapists, practitioners of aromatic medicine also give volatile oils by mouth. This sounds alarming and indeed it can be dangerous unless carried out in a controlled manner. Volatile oils should only be taken by mouth on the advice of an expert professional, although anyone who has eaten a cough sweet containing eucalyptus oil or a mint containing peppermint oil has taken pure volatile oils by mouth. Aromatic medicine is practised by medical doctors and herbalists to supplement their existing therapeutic options.

What are they good for?

Aromatherapists often use volatile oils to treat emotional and mental states such as anxiety, depression and irritability. The calming and uplifting effects of the scent of the oils are utilized by massage or inhalation. Relaxing oils give great results in relieving muscular tension and sedative oils can help with insomnia. Steam inhalation can ease sinus congestion and topical oil applications can treat skin infections such as ringworm (a fungal infection).

The use of volatile oils diffused as a room fragrance or employed in massage can confer valuable improvements when treating sexual disorders such as impotence and decreased libido. Digestive problems such as flatulence and indigestion can benefit from volatile oil treatment. Menstrual and menopausal problems can also be helped. Aromatic medicine covers much of the same area as aromatherapy but expands to include more serious disorders.

One particularly important area is the treatment of major infections. Volatile oils have antibacterial, antifungal and antiviral properties and can be effective against both external (skin) and internal infections. Aromatic medicine has a special role to play is in the treatment of chest infections.

Volatile oils offer vital potential in dealing with infective organisms that have become resistant to conventional antibiotic drugs.

Where does tree medicine fit in?

Many of the volatile oils used in aromatherapy and aromatic medicine are derived from trees, these include:

Abies species (fir trees) – Fir oil is made from the twigs and needles of several *Abies* trees. It is stimulating to the circulation and helps to generate heat and a vigorous state in the muscles. It is ideal in massages and baths for relieving muscular fatigue. It also disinfects the respiratory system, making it good as an inhalation or chest rub for head colds and chest infections.

Cananga odorata (ylang ylang) – The oil is prepared from the yellow flowers of this exotic tree. The common name means 'flower of flowers'. The scent is redolent of soap and commercial perfumes. It is used for depression, decreased sexual appetite, insomnia and high blood pressure.

Citrus aurantium (neroli) – Distilled from the flowers, neroli oil is one of the most delightful, and most expensive, of all the volatile oils. It is given for anxiety, depression, fatigue and for infections.

Cupressus sempervirens (cypress) – Obtained from the twigs and needles of cypress trees the oil is used to treat chest infections and general fatigue and debility. It has a particular value as an astringent for varicose veins and haemorrhoids.

Eucalyptus globulus (blue gum) – This is probably the best known and most widely used of the eucalyptus oils. It is prepared from the leaves and makes a first class antiseptic and decongestant in sinusitis and general infections of the upper respiratory tract.

Eucalyptus staigeriana (staigeriana) – This oil is also obtained from the leaves of a *Eucalyptus* species. In this case the oil has a very pleasant lemon scent and is useful for its sedative qualities.

Melaleuca leucadendron (cajuput) – This tree is a relative of the tea tree and its oil is distilled from the leaves. The oil has pain relieving properties and is antiseptic and antispasmodic. It has a wide range of uses from treating arthritic pain and gout through to easing bronchitis and colds.

Vitex agnus-castus (agnus castus) – The oil from the fruit of this Mediterranean tree is used to treat the symptoms of premenstrual syndrome (PMS). It is taken through the second half of the menstrual cycle as a cream applied to the thighs and abdomen.

How can I use them?

Many of the conditions that aromatherapists treat and the strategies they use are compatible with self-prescribed use at home – though you might need another person to help you out with the massage bit! Several adult education centres offer introductory courses. There are numerous books on the subject of varying quality, so browse through a well-stocked bookshop and choose a volume that appeals to you. Choose authors that have a professional qualification in aromatherapy and experience in practice. Professional training in aromatherapy typically takes two years as a part-time course.

Volatile oils are widely available, but be warned – the quality of these products is varied and many are very poor indeed. You should only buy from a reputable supplier. If possible, use organically grown oils. This is especially important with oils derived from fruit peel since these are often heavily sprayed with pesticides. Organic oils are expensive but remember that volatile oils are only used in drop doses and a little will go a long way. Below is a list of the various aromatherapy preparations and a description of how to use them:

Massage oils

Aromatherapy massage oils consist of a carrier oil (see Massage below) mixed with one or more volatile oils. The ratio of volatile oil to fixed oil can vary but in general it is advisable to stick to making the volatile oil content of massage oils in the region of 1–2%. This means that if you make up 100ml of massage oil you will use 1 or 2mls of volatile oils with 99 or 98mls of fixed oil. Volatile oils usually come in dropper bottles so it is important to know that 1ml is equivalent to 20 drops. You can make up oil blends in 100 or 200ml bottles for general use or make up a blend each time you massage. It is best to keep your mixes in glass bottles as these retain the properties of the oils better than plastic; volatile oils can also corrode plastic containers.

You can massage the whole body or just specific parts. Back, neck and shoulder massage is very popular as we store tremendous amounts of stress in this area, often leading to headaches. Massage of the hands and feet is tremendously relaxing. In children, for coughs and colds, it is best to massage over the sternum (breastbone) on the front of the chest, between the shoulder blades on the back and on the soles of the feet. A suitable massage blend for children's coughs and colds would be:

Eucalyptus smithii – 10 drops
Abies species – 10 drops
Sweet almond oil – 49ml

Add these together and store in a 50ml glass bottle. Apply to the child's sternum, back and feet 3–4 times a day, with the last massage on going to bed in the evening.

Most people will tolerate most volatile oils if properly diluted with a carrier oil. For children or people with sensitive skins patch test a small area of skin on the arm or leg to see if there is a reaction before massaging over a wider area. Face massage can be very soothing but use only highly diluted volatile oils because facial skin tends to be very sensitive. Always avoid volatile oils, even in diluted blends, coming into contact with the eyes, mouth and genitals.

Remember to cover prized bed linen with an old sheet or towels to avoid staining with oils and let oils fully absorb into the skin before dressing or they can ruin clothes.

Steam inhalation

Inhaling steam containing tiny droplets of volatile oils can be excellent for head colds and congested sinuses. Special inhalation applicators are available but are not essential. The method for an aromatic inhalation is as follows:

Boil a kettle of water and pour the just boiled water into a suitable container – large earthenware bowls are ideal. Leave the water to cool slightly for 2 minutes (using the water straight away can cause the oils to be too strong when inhaled). Then add 5–10 drops of volatile oil, just sprinkled on the surface of the water. Now place your head over the bowl at a safe distance and inhale for 5–10 minutes or until you feel you have had enough.

To increase the potency of an inhalation you can place a bath towel over your head and the bowl creating an enclosed steam chamber that will increase your exposure to the oils and retain the heat for longer. If you use the towel method it is good to cover your face with the towel as you move away from the steam and rest for a minute in this way before removing the towel completely. This makes for a gentler and more relaxing transition from hot steamy air to the cooler air in the room. A good blend for an inhalation for a head cold (blocked ears and sinuses) is:

> *Eucalyptus globulus* – 5 drops
> *Pinus* species – 5 drops

When the lining of the nose and throat is very inflamed, volatile oil inhalations can be irritating to the membranes, stop using inhalations if this occurs. Asthmatics may have their breathing problems exacerbated by inhalations and should use them with care. Children can benefit from inhalations but need constant supervision. An easy way to provide an inhalation for babies and small children, especially in emergencies, is to fill a sink with hot water, add the drops of volatile oils and hold the child carefully over the steam.

Creams

Volatile oils can be added to standard non-perfumed creams and then applied to the skin. Add volatile oils to the cream at the same ratio as for massage oils (1–2% volatile oil). For sinusitis you can add myrtle oil (*Myrtus communis*) to a cream and massage this either side of the nose. For varicose veins add cypress oil (*Cupressus sempervirens*), and for athlete's foot add tea tree oil (*Melaleuca alternifolia*).

Compresses

A compress is a warm water infusion that is soaked up into a cloth and then placed upon the skin on a particular body area. They are useful for treating painful or spasmodic muscular problems and bruises. To make an aromatic compress:

> Add 2–5 drops of volatile oils to 500ml(1 pint) of warm water.
>
> Mix together then place a cloth (a cotton tea towel or pillowcase is ideal) into the liquid. Soak the cloth thoroughly then wring it out until just damp, fold to size and place over the relevant area.

A good compress for period pain is to add 5 drops of ylang ylang oil (*Cananga odorata*) to 500ml of warm water and place the compress over the lower abdomen. The effectiveness of the compress can be increased by placing a hot-water bottle over it.

Baths

Volatile oils can be added to baths at a rate of 5–10 drops for a whole body bath, or 2–3 drops for a foot or hand bath. Mix the volatile oils with 5ml of a fixed oil such as almond oil before adding to the bath. Fir or pine oil baths are great for tired and stiff muscles, eucalyptus oil baths ease coughs and colds and petitgrain bigarade (*Citrus aurantium* leaf) added to a footbath taken just before going to bed is wonderful for sleep problems in children.

Flower waters

When volatile oils are distilled the oil section separates from the water-soluble fraction of the plant. The oil part is the volatile oil itself and the water part is known as flower water (also hydrosol or hydrolat). These waters retain some of the aromatic properties of the volatile oils but are weaker and therefore gentler. They can be very useful in therapy used as compresses or added to creams and baths. Some can be taken by mouth, diluted in water or juice.

Orange flower water (*Citrus aurantium* flowers) can be taken by mouth by children as a calming medicine for fractiousness and irritability. It is important to use only high-quality food grade flower waters and never to use cosmetic 'toilet waters'. Tree flower waters available from specialist suppliers include – tea tree, elder, juniper, laurel, pine, linden (*Tilia* species) and eucalyptus.

Cosmetics

Volatile oils can help to promote a healthy lifestyle by being incorporated into various cosmetic preparations. Floral waters make excellent make-up removers, volatile oils can be mixed with fixed oils to provide an alternative to shaving creams, and various oils can be used as ingredients in shampoos, perfumes, soaps, shower gels, moisturisers and many other cosmetic products.

Diffusion

Scenting the air in rooms with volatile oils can bring a number of benefits. Volatile oils naturally evaporate into the air but the process can be enhanced in several ways. Special volatile oil burners are available that usually consist of an evaporating dish placed over a nightlight candle, these need super-vision and safer (though much more expensive) electrical diffusers can be acquired. You can also use a lamp ring that clips around a light bulb and uses the light's heat to diffuse the oil or place the oils in a thin dish on top of a hot radiator.

You can use different blends for different purposes; for instance, to provide a sedative fragrance to treat sleeplessness, or to establish an erotic aroma to enhance sexual enjoyment and performance. A good blend to help provide an antiseptic and decongestant atmosphere for coughs and colds is:

Tea tree (*Melaleuca alternifolia*) – 2 drops
Pine (*Pinus sylvestris*) – 2 drops
Juniper (*Juniperus communis*) – 1 drop

Place this mixture in the diffuser and replace as it is exhausted.

FLOWER REMEDIES

What are they?

Healing flower remedies, or flower essences, are products made from plants that are used to treat the psychological rather than the physical state. They are essentially a kind of homeopathic preparation, being very dilute in terms of physical chemical content. They are made from herbaceous plants, shrubs and trees. The tree remedies are often prepared from the twigs as well as flowers. Most flower remedies are made in the following way:

- choose a clear sunny day and gather flowers from a particularly fine, and preferably wild, example of the desired plant;

- place the flowers immediately in a bowl of spring water in direct sunlight and next to the parent plant;

- leave to infuse in sunlight until the flowers wilt;

- add the infused water to brandy (as a preservative) – this is often in the ratio of one part infused water to 360 parts brandy.

This preparation is then ready to use and will store indefinitely. Several tree flower remedies are made in a different manner – by boiling the twigs and flowers in spring water before mixing with brandy.

The concept of flower remedies was developed by Dr Edward Bach (pronounced 'batch'). Born in 1886, he studied medicine in Birmingham and London and worked as a physician and bacteriologist. He was greatly influenced by the writings of the founding father of homeopathy Samuel

Hahnemann. In 1930 he retired from his post and devoted his time to developing a new system of medicine inspired by homeopathy but working on the personality traits and psychological characteristics of his patients rather than their physical symptoms. Over six years, until his death in 1936, he developed a set of 38 different remedies, of which 17 are derived from trees. He believed that this group of healing substances covered the entire spectrum of psychological states.

His way of choosing which plants had which properties was based on intuition rather than a rational scientific approach or a consideration of existing herbal traditional knowledge. A story relating to how Bach discovered the value of the red horse chestnut tree (*Aesculus* x *carnea*) illustrates his method. One day he was working outdoors when he cut his hand quite badly. This alarmed those around him but, looking beyond them into the distance, Bach saw a red horse chestnut tree in flower and realized that its flowers were the cure for the mental and emotional state he saw being acted out before him. That was it – red chestnut was the remedy for 'those who find it difficult not to be anxious for other people'. Such a technique of discovery has more to do with the mystic than the scientist and this pursuit of understanding through revelation gives powerful ammunition to the sceptic.

It may be that Dr Bach was a remarkable man with special abilities to read the book of nature but the question has to be asked – why should one person's impressions of the qualities of a particular plant be any more 'true' than another's? We all have different perceptions about the way plants feel to us; is it really possible to say which one is 'right'? Despite the questionable nature of their origins the Bach flower remedies are immensely popular today and many people feel that they are helped by the remedies. Bach himself wanted the flower remedies to be kept 'free from science, free from theories; for everything in Nature is simple'.

Although Bach considered his system complete, others have expanded his work, using the same kind of intuitive approach to find the qualities of other flowering plants. Australian naturopath Ian White developed the 'Australian Bush Flower Essences'. Prepared and taken in the same way as the Bach remedies they include plants such as the Illawarra flame tree (*Brachychiton acerifolius*). This flower remedy is given to those who experience a sense of rejection and it is said to instil feelings of confidence and self-approval. Other flower remedies include the 'Avalon Sentient Tree Essences' and 'Glastonbury Tree Essences'. The latter include willow, apple, yew and hawthorn.

What are they good for?

Flower remedies are used to treat our moods, thoughts and feelings, not our physical sensations. They can be used when the problem is entirely focused on emotional or mental levels or to treat the psychological aspects of a physical disease. They can be particularly useful in sensitive people who do not tolerate other medicines very well since flower remedies are very gentle and safe. These medicines are especially relevant in the treatment of chronic conditions that have a prominent degree of anxiety or psychological turmoil associated with them. Flower remedies may often be suitable in cases of chronic fatigue syndrome or ME.

They are suited to people experiencing particular worries, fears or negative patterns of behaviour. The 38 Bach flower remedies are divided into those that treat fear, uncertainty, lack of interest in present circumstances, loneliness, over-sensitivity to influences and ideas, despondency or despair and over-care for the welfare of others.

Working with flower remedies can be helpful for individuals who have set out upon a journey of personal discovery and growth. They are equally valuable in providing support when a process of change has been triggered in a more traumatic way, for instance, by divorce or bereavement. A compound flower remedy known as Rescue Remedy is given for shock and emergency states, it includes the tree cherry plum (*Prunus cerasifera*).

Where does tree medicine come in?

Many different plants are used in making flower remedies, trees included. Some flower remedy collections are based exclusively on trees. The trees used in the Bach remedies, and the reasons for their use, are:

Aspen – fear of unknown things

Beech – to develop greater tolerance and leniency in those who are overcritical or too strict

Cherry Plum – fear of losing control and doing things we might regret

Chestnut Bud – for people who fail to learn from their mistakes and therefore continue to make them

Crab Apple – a cleansing remedy for people who 'feel as if they had something not quite clean about themselves'

Elm – to support people who are seeking to achieve noble goals but who feel that the task they have set themselves is too difficult

Holly – for negative states such as jealousy and suspicion, for anger and irritation

Hornbeam – for those who are overwhelmed by everyday events and find it hard to carry on

Larch – for feelings of inadequacy and consequent lack of achievement

Oak – to support people who refuse to give in to illness or adverse life events and who battle on bravely, never giving up, though sometimes it would be better if they could rest and relax more and just 'go with the flow'

Olive – for those who are mentally and physically exhausted and feel they do not have enough strength to cope

Pine – for those who criticize and blame themselves

Red Chestnut – for anxiety about others

Sweet Chestnut – for moments of unbearable anguish when it seems that only oblivion awaits

Walnut – for times when we might be led astray by outside influences

White Chestnut – for repetitive unwanted thoughts

Willow – for those who are resentful of the hand that life has dealt them, who feel badly done by and tend to complain a lot

How can I use them?

Dr Bach envisioned that flower remedies would be self-prescribed, they would truly be the people's medicine, not requiring the intercession of a practitioner. Practitioner courses are now available but they are not really necessary. The principles of flower remedy therapy are basic and easy to grasp. Since the remedies themselves are very safe and because they offer psychological support rather than physical treatment they are, as Bach asserted, ideally suited for self-use.

If you are interested in using these medicines for yourself or family, the best place to start is with the original flower remedies. Dr Bach's book, *The Twelve Healers and Other Remedies*, is still in print and provides all you really need to know to begin using the remedies in one slim volume. Simply read through the descriptions of each remedy and decide which ones apply to you. Then take the specific remedy as a couple of drops on the tongue or in water. If you find it difficult to analyse your own state then ask a trusted friend to select the remedy for you.

Herbal Medicine

What is it?

Herbal medicine is the use of whole plant preparations to promote health and to prevent or treat disease. Herbal remedies are made from roots, barks, leaves, flowers, fruits and seeds, either singly or in combinations. The remedies are minimally processed thereby retaining a full range of the plants' original constituents. Herbalists contend that this makes herbal medicines safer than purified conventional drugs. The herbalist's approach is naturopathic (working with, rather than against, nature) and holistic (the herbal practitioner aims to use the whole plant to treat the whole person).

Herbal medicine is the oldest of all medical systems and conventional Western medicine evolved out of herbalism. Today the word 'phytotherapy' (from the Greek *phyto*, meaning plant) is sometimes used to describe the professional practice of a scientific rational approach to plant therapeutics. There are a number of different herbal approaches including Western herbal medicine (based on a modern scientific medical perspective), traditional Chinese herbal medicine, Ayurvedic medicine and Kanpo (traditional Japanese medicine). Modern herbal medicine combines sound traditional knowledge with the latest research findings and today's practitioners aim to combine both the art and the science of medicine.

Although many herbs can be self-prescribed for home use, some herbs are very powerful and need to be used with great care. A qualified herbal practitioner will prescribe the more potent herbs. Although high-quality modern herbalism in the Western approach is hard to find outside of countries such as the UK and Australia, most countries have their own traditional herbal healers. The practice of traditional herbalism is particularly sophisticated in countries such as China, India and Africa. In the USA legislation varies between states but in many the practice of herbalism is prohibited. Similarly, in France it is only possible to diagnose and treat disease if you are a qualified medical doctor. However, many conventional doctors in France and Germany do prescribe herbs for their patients.

A first consultation with a Western herbalist will normally take around one hour. The herbalist will take a detailed case history paying attention to all aspects of your health from birth onwards and looking at your diet, work and lifestyle. Then the herbalist will carry out any relevant physical examination and refer you for further tests if they are required. Professional herbal treatment will involve advice on diet and lifestyle factors as well as the prescription of herbal medicines.

What is it good for?

Herbal medicines can treat the majority of conditions that you might consult your doctor about. Conditions that are clearly not susceptible to herbal treatment include insulin-dependent diabetes and serious infective disorders such as meningitis. Most conditions requiring treatment in hospital can only be helped to a limited extent by herbal medicine. Problems that can generally benefit to a significant degree from herbal medicines include:

Digestive – constipation, flatulence, indigestion, irritable bowel;

Gynaecological – menstrual problems, menopausal symptoms;

Heart and circulation – angina, high blood pressure, varicose veins;

Joints and muscles – arthritis, muscular pain;

Nervous system – headaches, migraine, depression, anxiety;

Respiratory – asthma, hay fever, bronchitis, coughs;

Skin – acne, eczema, psoriasis, fungal infections.

Herbs can help with many infections such as influenza, and with immune system problems (autoimmune illnesses and decreased immune functioning), and offer tremendous support in dealing with the effects of stress and tension.

Where does tree medicine fit in?

Herbal medicine uses all types of plants but trees provide a significant proportion of herbal remedies. The tree profiles in Part II of this book give many examples of the use of trees in herbal medicine.

How can I use it?

When using herbs at home it is important to stay with those that are known to be well tolerated and safe. A wide variety of herbs can be safely and effectively self-prescribed after studying one of the many good books on herbs that are available. Try and use books that have been written by qualified and experienced herbalists. It is preferable to buy herbs rather than to collect them from the wild. Collecting herbs from the wild depletes natural populations and it can also be dangerous if you misidentify plants. Never collect any plant, from the wild or the garden, unless you are absolutely certain that you know what it is. An alternative is to grow herbs yourself from certified seed.

When treating children, the elderly and when pregnant or breastfeeding, herbs should always be used with particular care and usually at a lower dosage. It is not advisable to take herbs in pregnancy unless on the advice of an expert professional herbalist. If you are taking prescribed conventional medicines you should consult your doctor or a qualified herbalist before starting a course of herbal treatment since some herbs can interfere with drug actions. Below are listed the various types of herbal preparations and the ways in which they can be used.

Tea

Herbal teas can be made in two ways, by infusion or decoction. Infusions, sometimes called tisanes, are made by covering herbs with hot water and leaving the mixture to brew before using, much in the same way as you would make a cup of China or Indian tea. This method is suitable for soft plant tissues such as leaves, flowers and fine seeds.

Decoctions are made by simmering herbs in water, in order to release the constituents contained within hard plant tissues such as roots, barks, waxy leaves, fruits and seeds. Before decocting hard plant parts, it helps to crush them in a pestle and mortar first. Decoction is not recommended for plant parts that contain a lot of volatile oils as they tend to evaporate away during the process.

To make an infusion:

> Pour 250ml (a mugful) of just boiled water over 2–3 teaspoons of the herbs, cover over and leave to brew for 5 minutes, then stir, strain and drink. Take the tea 2–4 times a day. You can brew herbs in a teapot or in a mug with a saucer over the top.

To make a decoction:

> Place 2–3 teaspoons of the herbs in a non-aluminium pan (stainless steel or enamel are ideal), pour on 300ml of water and simmer gently for 10 minutes. Then stir, strain and drink. Take the decoction 2–4 times a day.

To avoid having to make your infusion or decoction several times each day you can make up 2–4 cups all at the same time, drink one cup and pour the rest into a thermos flask for use later in the day. This is especially useful if you are at work or on the move.

Tincture

Tinctures are liquid herbal medicines made by brewing herbs in an alcohol and water solution. The amount of alcohol varies depending on the constituents in the plants. Herbs with largely water-soluble components are made at 25% alcohol. Those with a high volatile oil content (such as cloves) need around 45% alcohol to extract them optimally while resin containing plants (such as myrrh) need a very high alcohol content of 90%. The ratio of herb to fluid also varies but in general a standard tincture is made at 1:5 (1 part herb to every 5 parts of alcohol/water fluid) this works out as 200g (7oz) of herb in every 1 litre of tincture. Many professional herbalists use stronger tinctures of 1:2 (500g (17½oz) in every litre) or 1:1 (where the tincture works out as 1 kilo of herb to a litre).

Dosage varies depending on the strength of the tincture and the herb used but a standard adult dose for a mixture of basic 1:5 tinctures is 5ml (1 teaspoon) taken three times a day. Tinctures should always be taken in a glass of water or juice.

Tinctures have a long shelf-life and last almost indefinitely. They are normally assumed to be active for at least 2–3 years.

Creams and ointments

Ointments are fatty preparations that do not contain water and are poorly absorbed by the skin; they form a greasy layer over it. Creams are a mixture of water and fats that form a soft layer that mixes with skin and is absorbed by it.

Herbal creams and ointments start with a suitable base cream or ointment preparation to which herbal preparations are added. Dried herbs are mixed with the base and heated together in a bain marie or slow cooker for around 2–3 hours then strained; the liquefied herb-infused base is left to set into a solid cream or ointment. Base materials can also have infused oils (*see* below) or tinctures added to them to make herbal creams.

A good cream to use for chapped lips and hands, and to apply over congested sinuses, is made as follows:

> Put 50g of a simple non-perfumed base cream into a bowl; add 5ml of infused elderflower oil and 5ml of infused limeflower oil and mix together thoroughly. (You can add 4 drops of benzoin tincture as a preservative but this is optional.) Put into a jar and use as required.

A cream such as this will keep for 6–12 months. Keep it in a cool dark place or in the fridge.

Syrup

Syrups are made by combining infusions or decoctions with unrefined sugar.

> Make up 500ml (1 pint) of an infusion or decoction of your chosen herb and mix this in a non-aluminium saucepan with 500g (17½oz) of unrefined sugar (you can use an equal amount of runny honey instead). Simmer the mixture very gently to avoid burning the sugar until the mixture takes on the consistency of a thick syrup. Then turn off the heat and allow the mixture to cool completely. Now pour the syrup into a dark glass bottle and seal with a cork stopper. Take 1–2 teaspoons (5–10ml) as required either neat or in a little water or juice.

Syrups are soothing due to the demulcent effect of the sugars coating the membranes of the throat and oesophagus. They also taste nice! This can help to persuade children to take herbal medicines. Many syrups are used as cough medicines, this is mainly due to the soothing effects of the sugars on inflamed throats. One of the best cough syrups is made with wild cherry bark (*Prunus serotina*); it has a delicious aniseed taste.

Juice

Juices are made by pressing succulent fresh plant parts such as some leaves, flowers, fruits and seeds. They should be drunk fresh unless a preservative is added. Fresh tree fruit juices are tremendously energizing and can be taken as part of your everyday diet. Other juices are used as specific medicines. Tree juices include acerola cherries (rich in vitamin C), birch leaves, ginkgo leaves, hawthorn flowers and leaves and juniper berries. Elderberry juice is a fantastic treatment for colds and influenza.

Infused oil

Infused oils are made by adding plant parts to a cold-pressed fixed oil, such as almond oil, leaving the mixture to macerate, and then straining the infused oil. A hot infusion is used for extracting leaves:

> Infuse the warmed oil and herb mixture in a bain marie (a glass bowl over a pan of simmering water will do fine) for 3–4 hours.

A cold infusion is used for flowers:

> Pour the fixed oil over a large glass jar full of the required flowers until they are completely covered then seal and leave to infuse for 2–4 weeks.

Once infused, strain the oil through a muslin bag and store in a dark bottle in a cool dark place. The oil will keep for 6–12 months. Infused oils can be added to creams and ointments or used as they are as massage oils. Lime-flower infused oil is wonderfully soothing and healing to dry or flaky skin.

Tablets and capsules

Tablets and capsules are convenient ways to take herbal medicines but they are not always as effective as preparations such as teas and tinctures. They are made either from powdered dried herbs or from liquid preparations that have been spray dried. It is often difficult to get enough herbal content into tablets and capsules in terms of the sheer volume of herbal material that is required to have a significant therapeutic effect. For this reason the more concentrated high-potency tablets are to be preferred, although this does depend on the strength of the particular herb concerned.

Slippery elm (*Ulmus rubra*) tablets are excellent for treating digestive problems such as heartburn, stomach irritation and ulceration, indigestion and diverticulitis. The tablets are made from compacted slippery elm powder that swells up as it moves along the digestive system, coating the linings of the digestive tract in a soothing and nutritious gel. To treat irritable digestive problems take 2 standard slippery elm tablets before each meal. Make sure that you wash the tablets down with 2–3 glasses of water to provide the fluid that the tablets require in order to swell up effectively.

Compress

Compresses have been described under aromatherapy above. Herbal compresses are made by soaking a cloth in an infusion or decoction of the required herb, wringing it out and then applying it to the affected area.

A compress made with a decoction of witch hazel (*Hamamelis virginiana*) bark is very helpful when applied to bruises or sprained ankles.

Poultice

A poultice is similar to a compress but, instead of applying an infusion or decoction of the herb to the skin, you apply the herb itself. It can be made with dried or fresh herbs and is usually applied warm. A poultice of powdered slippery elm bark has been traditionally used as a drawing agent. It helps to soften and swell the skin making it easier to extract foreign bodies such as thorns or splinters. It also helps to bring painful boils to a head. To make a slippery elm poultice:

Mix 100g of the powder with sufficient water to form a thick paste, then pack the paste over the affected area and hold in place with a piece of cloth. Leave on for about 15 minutes or until the desired effects are achieved.

Gargle and mouthwash

Gargles and mouthwashes are prepared from infusions, decoctions or tinctures. Simply prepare the required tea or dilute the tincture with water and use. For a gargle use a cup of tea or 5ml of tincture in a cup of water and gargle with sips of the liquid. Take a sip, gargle, spit the fluid out then take another sip and repeat again. Continue to do this for about 5 minutes until the liquid has all been used up. Use the same amounts of liquid for a mouthwash and swill sips of the fluid around the mouth, flushing it around the tongue, teeth and gums repeatedly. A good mixture for mouth and throat infections is made by blending the following tinctures:

Myrrh (*Commiphora molmol*) – 20ml
Clove (*Syzygium aromaticum*) – 30ml
Pau d'arco (*Tabebuia species*) – 50ml

This makes 100ml of tincture. Use 5ml at a time diluted in a glass of water.

Baths

Herbal baths are made by adding infusions or decoctions to bath water or by infusing sachets of herbs in the bath water itself. For a full bath, use about 100g (3½oz) of herb, with half that amount for foot or hand baths. Pine needle baths are good for muscular pains, arthritis and rheumatism and lime flower baths are good for settling fractious or feverish children.

Footbaths are excellent at the end of a long day to ease tired feet but they can also have more widespread effects. They are particularly useful for children who refuse to take herbs by mouth. Adults with sweaty feet can try oak bark footbaths.

Herbal handbaths can help to relieve the tension that builds up in the muscles of the hands, particularly in those who use their hands intensively for a living such as typists and factory machine operators. A decoction made from willow bark and black haw (*Viburnum prunifolium*) bark added to a suitable bowl full of warm water makes a useful handbath for arthritic and muscular hand pains and repetitive strain injuries.

Eyebath

Eyebaths are used for conditions such as inflammation (conjunctivitis) and production of excessive mucous. They can be useful in eye infections and allergic conditions such as hay fever where the eyes become sore and irritable. To make an eyebath:

> Prepare an infusion or decoction of the required herb. Strain the liquid from the herb very thoroughly, ensuring that there are no plant particles left in the fluid as these may irritate the eye. Let the tea become lukewarm then pour into a plastic eyebath. Lean forward and place the eyebath closely beneath the eye, now straighten up and lean backwards allowing the contents of the bath to tip over the eye blinking a few times. Use a different eyebath for each eye to avoid cross-contamination.

You can also make an eyebath using tinctures. Add 1–2 drops of tincture to an eyebath containing cooled boiled water and proceed as above. For sore eyes it is good to soak 2 cotton wool pads with the desired tea or tincture/water mixture and place these over closed eyes. Rest for 5–10 minutes with the eyes closed and the soothing herbs relieving the soreness. A suitable herb for making such a soothing application is elderflowers.

Pessaries and suppositories

Pessaries and suppositories are bullet-shaped and are made out of solidified fats such as cocoa butter. The fats are mixed with herbal preparations such as teas or tinctures before setting. The fats melt at body temperature and thereby release their therapeutic constituents when inserted into the body.

Pessaries are inserted into the vagina and can be used to treat thrush and persistent discharges (leucorrhoea). Myrrh tincture can be incorporated to treat thrush and oak bark pessaries are useful for leucorrhoea.

Suppositories are inserted into the anus and are a good way of treating piles or irritation. Witch hazel and horse chestnut suppositories are good for piles.

MASSAGE

What is it?

Massage is the manipulation of the body's soft tissues (skin and muscles) to promote healthy physical functioning of the body and to treat pain and discomfort in the body's tissues and organs. When we feel an itch we scratch it, if an area of skin is cold or sore we rub it and if our muscles are stiff we squeeze them. These are all instinctive forms of massage. Many of us are very good at massaging ourselves, our partners and our children, without any training at all. We instinctively know how to touch others in a natural and positive way. Some people are more comfortable with this than others. We all express ourselves and learn new things in different ways – some people tend to interact with the world in a primarily visual way, others are particularly sensitive to sound, taste or smell. For those of us who have a pronounced sense of touch, massage is often something of a natural talent.

There are a number of specific systems of massage. Many cultures have their own indigenous forms of massage therapy, some of which go beyond muscular movement into joint manipulation. Thai massage, for instance, involves a dynamic physical encounter between patient and therapist where the practitioner not only uses their hands but also elbows, knees and feet to take the patient through a series of pronounced stretching movements. We tend to think of massage as being a type of relaxation therapy but it can also be very stimulating and enervating. Brisk massage tends to bring a wave of strong circulatory activity around the body and is very refreshing and awakening. Deep tissue massage can release a lot of stored waste products of metabolism, or 'toxins', into the circulation initially. This is an area for professional therapists since there is potential to harm tissues and organs with deep pressure and the side effects of 'toxin release' can be unpleasant – including headaches, skin rashes, fatigue and nausea. Slow and gentle massage is the best option for non-practitioner use and it can be very soothing, helping to release built-up stress and tension.

The most commonly practised type of massage is Swedish massage. This is based on a scientific understanding of anatomy and physiology and uses three main techniques. These are 'effleurage' (gentle stroking movements), 'petrissage' (deeper penetrating movements) and 'tapotement' (specific movements such as chopping, thumb pressure and cupping – using cupped hands in rapid stimulating movements).

What is it good for?

Massage is great for relieving muscular tension due to stress – countering the consequences of overworking the mind and body. It can help with tension headaches, stomachaches and period pain. By improving general blood flow, thereby enhancing the oxygenation and nutrition of tissues, it can have far-reaching effects, assisting a large number of physical and some psychological problems.

Where does tree medicine fit in?

The connection between trees and massage is in the use of tree fixed oils (as lubricants and healing balms) to act as an interface between the practitioner's hands and the patient's body. Tree oils are necessary to reduce friction when massaging and they also nourish and heal the skin. The oils make it possible to generate heat in the skin and muscles, thus promoting relaxation and suppleness.

A number of tree oils can be used including avocado, apricot kernel, peach kernel, hazelnut and walnut. Sweet almond oil is perhaps the most commonly used massage oil and it is delightfully light and pleasant to handle. Alexandrian laurel or tamanu (*Calophyllum inophyllum*) yields an oil that is calming and warming. The oil is pressed from the seeds of this Malaysian tree and contains chemicals (inophyllums, a type of coumarin) that show activity against HIV (they block the reverse transcriptase mechanism that is crucial in HIV development). It is also nutritionally rich in proteins.

Another interesting oil is andiroba from the large South American tree

Carapa guianensis. Again, the oil is pressed from the trees seeds (nuts). It was once used to mummify human heads collected in battle! Nowadays it is more prized for its anti-imflammatory qualities – it is excellent for massaging sore muscles and around arthritic joints. It can also be applied to areas of bruising, eczema, psoriaisis and over small healing wounds.

How can I use it?

One of the great things about massage is that anyone can do it. We all have access to an instinctive knowledge of how to use our hands to touch others. This can be expressed in a sexual way but we constantly use other forms of touch – when meeting people we shake hands, when comforting friends we put our arms around them, when our children are ill we smooth their brows. Using massage at home for friends and family can be very rewarding. It's great to take it in turns with a partner to give and receive a massage at the end of the day to relax and unwind. When children have stomachaches a gentle circular clockwise massage of the abdomen can be very soothing.

Intimate massage can be a form of 'sexual healing' with tree oils providing a sensuous medium between partners. Many cases of male impotence and lowered sexual appetite in both sexes are due to fatigue or anxiety. Intimate massage accompanied by candlelight and gentle music can be a wonderful way to arouse sexual energy and confidence.

There are a number of good illustrated books that can demonstrate useful massage routines but it is an art that ideally needs to be taught in person. Many adult education centres provide introductory classes in massage that are excellent for learning the basic principles. Why not attend with a friend or partner – you can then exchange massages and help keep each other relaxed and healthy? Specialist classes in baby massage are also available for parents and carers. If you can't get to classes then instructional videos can be the next best thing.

Massage can be applied to the whole body or to specific parts. The back and neck are the most commonly massaged regions of the body but individual massage of the hands, feet or face is particularly relaxing – we tend to forget how much tension is held in these areas. Indian head massage is another practice that is becoming increasingly popular.

If you are unsure about whether massage is for you then the best way to find out is to visit a professional massage therapist for treatment. Massage sessions can last anything from half an hour to two hours depending on the type of massage and the area of the body covered. It is good, at least on initial visits, to organize things so that you can go home and rest or sleep after a treatment as it can make you feel quite tired. Ideally, have a bath after your massage and then sleep. This will reinforce the healing and relaxing effects of the therapy. It's great to fit in a massage session once a week, even if you don't have any particular muscular problems, as part of a healthy living routine.

MEDITATION AND VISUALIZATION

What are they?

Meditation can be defined in many ways; the everyday meaning of the word is 'to reflect or contemplate', but the dedicated practice of meditation goes beyond this. Meditation, as a specific discipline, is a form of mental exercise that helps practitioners forge a contact with the dimensions of the spirit or soul. On this level it is considered to be possible to develop a clearer understanding of issues, to gain an insight into the greater picture and discover how to proceed ahead in the most positive and productive manner. Meditation is a way of achieving spiritual union in a mystical or religious sense, and is also used by people with no specific faith. In many Eastern countries it is an everyday practice analogous to the Christian ritual of prayer.

There are several schools of thought in meditation and a major common theme is the use of meditation as a constructive problem-solving technique. Here, the purpose of meditation is to form a bridge from the current situation to an improved future. In meditation we can take a current area of interest and concern, formulate a question about it and meditate on finding an answer. This issue need not be a personal one; it could be about a matter of global significance. During the meditation the experience can be likened to turning the issue into a jewel, holding it to the light and considering its every facet and dimension. On completion we may have gained a fuller understanding of the issue and be able to proceed to apply the insights we have received.

Visualization is often confused with meditation and it can be viewed as one aspect of it. Visualization is a way of applying thought to achieve a concrete effect. It is a way of creating an image and imbuing it with detail in the belief that it will become 'real'. This practice is based on the esoteric principle that 'energy follows thought'.

What are they good for?

It is often thought that meditation is about achieving 'inner peace'. This can be the case but it is an active way of pursuing peace, a peace that is achieved through confronting and considering issues rather than escaping from them. Meditation is a way of gaining insight, vision and control. It is empowering, energizing and restorative. It can promote a sense of equilibrium – a balance between the physical, emotional, mental and spiritual bodies. In fact, meditation should be seen as a type of mental and spiritual activity that supplements and complements physical exercise and emotional responses. In short it helps to round us out as individuals, to make us more complete, more integrated and whole.

When we feel a lack of vision, meaning and purpose, meditation can help us find new ways of looking at things and provide new options and ideas. Once established as a regular practice it can be used daily to review where we are at in our lives and to plan our next moves. With consistent use, meditation promotes mental and spiritual health just as surely as regular swimming or cycling engenders our physical health.

Visualization can be used when we are unwell to imagine ourselves becoming better in the belief that where the mind leads the body will follow. Clearly, there are limitations to this practice. It would be unreasonable to suggest that everyone can just 'think themselves well'. It would also be wrong to suggest that visualization can replace other types of medical treatment. However there is certainly a role for this method to complement other therapies and many healers use visualization to treat their patients. Some healers focus energy on certain areas of the body and visualize the changes taking place in that area. This can be quite general, for instance visualizing an area being suffused with a bright cleansing light, or very specific, such as imagining an increase in healthy white blood cells destroying an area of infection.

Visualizations have been part of the regime at the Bristol Cancer Centre in England for many years and many patients have found it helpful. There is no doubt that visualization can help people to feel that they have an influence over their health and are not merely victims of it. This sense of control can be tremendously positive and improve a person's quality of life.

Where does tree medicine fit in?

You could be forgiven, at this stage, for thinking – very interesting but what has this all got to do with trees? The answer is that both meditation and visualization often work with specific powerful images and trees are commonly used as a focus for thought.

Meditation needs to be structured and focused in order to be effective. Focussing on images or concepts or questions helps to produce a useful, productive meditative experience. In Tibetan meditation the image of the Buddha or other great spiritual leaders is used as a 'jumping-off point' to explore wider concepts. Natural images are also used, foremost amongst these being the tree. In meditation the tree is often seen as a living organism connecting the physical and the spiritual, earth and heaven. Trees can be experienced as a link between the mundane and the divine – contemplation of the various aspects of this relationship can leave one with an enhanced sense of connection with nature and imbues everyday experience with a sense of the sacred.

When meditating upon the image of a tree, it may be that we see it as actually breathing, inhaling pollution and exhaling shimmering clean air. There can also be a connection with the view of nature as a living being, something we are all intimately part of. Such insights can lead to a renewed dedication to protect the environment and honour this perception of a vital interdependence. The whole experience can be regenerative and deeply moving. In visualization, tree images can be developed as metaphors for our own feelings of health and well-being. We can imagine ourselves drawing strength, or gracefulness, or whatever the particular quality we desire may be, from a particular tree.

How can I use them?

The popular image of a person meditating is of someone sitting cross-legged on the floor with their eyes closed and a blissful expression on their face. In fact, when meditating you can sit in any position you find comfortable. Many people find it easier to close their eyes but in some practices, such as certain Tibetan traditions, meditation is performed with the eyes open. In practice, just be yourself and do what feels most natural to you. Meditation is an everyday practice open to everyone. It is about finding clarity and understanding, not necessarily attaining nirvana.

Too often novices sit blankly waiting for inspiration and are disheartened when nothing arrives. Meditation needs to be more disciplined and focused to be worthwhile. When meditating using trees as images, start with a specific image in mind. This may be a photograph, a memory, or an imagined picture of a tree or trees. Have a specific question in mind before you meditate such as "What can I learn from this tree?'; 'What is the purpose of this forest?'; 'How can trees heal?'; 'How can I work with trees?' You may wish to explore a particular cultural or historical idea such as the concept of the 'world tree' or the 'healing tree'. A question could be 'I would like to explore the world tree, what does this mean?' You might start with an image of the world tree gathered from a particular traditional image or description.

Meditate in quiet and comfortable surroundings, the temperature should be neither too cold nor too hot. You can meditate indoors or outdoors but it helps to relax if you can be sure that you will not be interrupted. Assume a comfortable position and focus your attention on the mental plane. It can help to say and imagine the following – 'Relax the physical body, quiet the emotional body, steady the mind'. Repeat this until you feel calm and settled, ready to consider and think. Then bring your tree image and your question forward in your mind; follow your train of thought and the images that arise until you feel a sense of conclusion.

When coming out of meditation refocus yourself on the physical plane and spend a little time consolidating before getting on with other things. Such a meditation should last only 5–10 minutes, more extended meditation can be very tiring. It is often helpful to return to the same image or idea on several occasions to explore it fully and gain a clear understanding of what it holds.

There are a number of meditation courses available either by attendance at classes or by home learning. Have a look at the available options and find out which approach appeals to you.

Visualization can begin in a similar way to meditation but the emphasis is on associating with a particular concept via a meaningful image. Trees may be used in visualization to engender the development of certain qualities and attributes. For example, you can visualize an image of an oak tree, focusing on its strength, and then associate that strength with yourself. This can be reinforced by repetition of words such as, 'I am strong like the oak', to help imbue oneself with the desired qualities. In the same way, you could visualize the grace of the birch, the endurance of the yew or the vigour of pines.

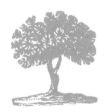

NUTRITIONAL MEDICINE

What is it?

The role of nutrition in healthcare is often overlooked by conventional medicine. Although dieticians have an important role to play it is often a limited one, focusing on the nutritional aspects of only a few diseases such as diabetes. There is a lack of a sense that nutrition plays a pivotal role in everybody's health.

Nutritional medicine works with our food intake, boosted by nutritional supplements where appropriate, to promote optimum health and to prevent and help treat disease. It acknowledges that good nutrition is one of the central pillars of good health, along with activity and rest, on each of the physical, emotional, mental and spiritual levels. We cannot live without eating and the quality of our lives depends to a large extent on the quality of our diets. In the West we are living longer but the quality of lives in our later years sometimes leaves much to be desired. As we age, the consequences of a high fat and sugar diet catches up with us in the form of heart disease and late onset diabetes. Obesity is a major problem and it is becoming more prevalent in younger people.

While nutrition has a great contribution to make towards recovering from illness, it is much more effective as a means of prevention. Dietary requirements vary between individuals depending on sex, weight, energy demands, whether pregnant or lactating and so on. A nutritionist can advise upon what is the diet that best meets individual requirements. Nonetheless there are some basic rules you can work with:

- match calorie intake to energy output; that is to say, you can eat more if you are being very physically active and less if you are not;

- avoid taking foods that can prevent absorption of nutrients – such as strong China or Indian tea;

- do not smoke;

- keep to a moderate alcohol intake – there is evidence that moderate red wine and whisky intake can even have some beneficial effects;

- eat complex rather than refined carbohydrates – do have wholemeal bread, pasta, rice and beans, but avoid white flour products and sugar;

- avoid saturated fats such as animal fats and avoid fried food in general;

- supplement your diet with essential fatty acids rich in omega 3 fats – such as flax oil and hemp oil (about a teaspoon of oil a day for the average adult);

- eat oily fish (such as mackerel, herrings) and chicken rather than red meat;

- keep to a high fruit and vegetable intake – eat at least 5 servings a day (this does not include potatoes);

- eat nuts and seeds regularly (pumpkin and sunflower seeds are excellent);

- drink 1–2 litres of pure water a day and avoid fizzy drinks, substitute herb teas for tea and coffee (rooibosch (red bush) tea and roasted dandelion root coffee).

What is it good for?

The potential benefits, economic and otherwise, of a healthy nation are beginning to be understood by governments. The old adage about prevention being better than cure is starting to be applied. In the UK there have been plans to launch health advisory centres in towns that will provide the opportunity for anyone to call in and ask about what can be done to improve their diet and general health. Such centres will conduct tests such as for blood pressure and cholesterol, aiming to catch problems before they start or at an early stage when more can be easily done to halt the progress of disease.

In addition to disease prevention, and the treatment of heart disease and diabetes, nutritional medicine is thought to have a part to play in controlling and relieving several other disorders. Too much of the wrong food (dietary excess) or too little of the right food (nutritional deficiencies) can contribute to anaemia, anxiety and other mood disorders, asthma, some cancers, eczema, fatigue, headaches, menstrual and menopausal problems and a host of other conditions.

Perhaps the main benefit of nutritional medicine is that it can help us to achieve a diet that enables us to fulfil our potential. Being well nourished, in the sense of being properly rather than excessively fed, makes us feel energetic, positive, calm, considered and capable. It sets the foundations for us to get on and do what we want to with our lives. Many of the physical and mood disorders that hold us back can be alleviated if we are prepared to change our diets. A good nutritionist can help us to achieve this. A transformation in well-being can occur from relatively simple measures such as eliminating caffeine from the diet and ensuring adequate intake of basic essential fatty acids, vitamins, minerals and trace nutrients.

Where does tree medicine fit in?

Trees are a major source of the nutrients we need. They provide us with many of our most healthy and important nutritional substances all wrapped up in tasty, attractive and accessible packages! While there is a thriving industry in nutritional supplements (food chemicals in pills), it remains important for us to take our nutrients in their original state.

Herbalists believe that medicinal plants are usually safer and more gently effective when taken as a whole, rather than when individual chemicals are extracted from them as purified constituents. The herbalist contends that there are numerous cofactors in the whole plant that make it better absorbed, assist it in having its beneficial effects and help prevent side effects. While purified nutritional components of plants do not have the same potential for harm as conventional drugs derived from herbs, it is still the case that they are often less well absorbed and less effective than when they are taken as part of an actual food.

There is an argument that our soils are less nutritionally rich than they were in the past and that consequently it is hard for us to get all our nutritional requirements from the traditional method of just eating food. This should not be the case for certified organically grown foods. Below is a summary of how trees can help us to stay in good health through our use of them in the daily diet:

Balancing fats

Some fats are bad (such as LDL cholesterol and triglycerides) and others are good (such as omega 3 and 6 essential fatty acids). We need to encourage the good fats and discourage the bad ones. Olive oil is rich in monounsaturated fats, which are well-known to decrease the amount of unhealthy saturated fats in the body and protect the arteries and the heart. Avocados are another good source of monounsaturated fatty acids and a trial has shown that they can reduce cholesterol levels.

A large study, involving nearly 800 people, males and females from 18–65 years of age, looked at the effects of eating walnuts on cholesterol levels. The researchers found that levels of the healthy HDL cholesterol rose in those subjects who regularly ate walnuts – this type of cholesterol is associated with a lower risk of heart disease. Pectins from fruit skins are a source of high quality soluble fibre that binds to cholesterol and removes it from the body. This type of fibre is less well-known than bran roughage but in fact it is more effective at lowering cholesterol and it is gentler on the bowel.

Providing vitamins, minerals and trace elements

Vitamins

Vitamin A – This vitamin is not found in vegetable materials but its precursors, the carotenes, are. Upon eating carotenes, which give the yellow and orange colours to fruits and vegetables, they are converted to vitamin A. Beta-carotene is the best known and most valuable of the carotenes and is present in fruits such as apricots and mangoes. Another carotene called lycopene is present in high amounts in guavas (the richest source is tomatoes).

Vitamin A is essential for good night vision and healthy skin. It can cause problems when taken in excess, especially in pregnant women where it has been associated with birth defects. Pregnant women should avoid vitamin A supplements and excessively rich sources of this nutrient such as liver but there is no need to be concerned about carotene intake in fruits since these are only present at relatively low levels.

B vitamins – This group of vitamins has numerous uses, mainly mediated by influencing enzyme functions.

- **Vitamin B1** (thiamin) is found in fruits such as oranges and in nuts such as pine nuts, Brazil nuts, pecans, hazelnuts and cashews. Deficiency causes the disease beriberi – this is rare in the developed world except in alcoholics. Mild deficiency has been associated with fatigue and depression.

- **Vitamin B2** (riboflavin) is involved in energy production and the regeneration of glutathione that protects against free-radical damage to cells. Deficiency causes cracking at the corners of the mouth (angular stomatitis), red tongue and visual disturbances; it is also associated with the common skin disorder seborrhoeic dermatitis. Vitamin B2 is present in nuts such as almonds.

- **Niacin** is classed as a B vitamin (sometimes called vitamin B3) and is present in moderate amounts in nuts including pine nuts and almonds. Deficiency causes the disease pellagra. In the diet it is helpful in controlling blood sugar and cholesterol levels.

- **Vitamin B6** (pyridoxine) has been associated with improving the symptoms of premenstrual syndrome and can be obtained from fruits such as oranges and avocados, and nuts including walnuts, hazelnuts and chestnuts.

- **Folic acid** works alongside vitamin B12 in controlling cell division and it is essential in helping to prevent certain neurological conditions such as spina bifida developing in early pregnancy. It is obtained most abundantly from green leafy vegetables but is also present in moderate amounts in fruits (such as oranges) and nuts (such as almonds, walnuts).

- **Pantothenic acid** (sometimes called vitamin B5) is needed to facilitate the release of energy from fats and carbohydrates. It is present in most foods so deficiency is rare – its name is derived from the Greek *pantos* meaning 'everywhere'. It is particularly abundant in nuts such as pecans and cashews and in avocados.

- **Biotin** is involved in fat metabolism and only small amounts are required, it can be obtained from many nuts such as walnuts, pecans and almonds. It is also manufactured in the intestines, especially by vegetarians.

Vitamin C (ascorbic acid) – This is essential to maintain strong and healthy connective tissue. Deficiency causes bleeding into the skin and from the gums. It is also important in stimulating defence against infection via the immune system.

Vitamin C is sensitive to exposure to the air and heat so is best obtained from fresh uncooked foods. It can be obtained from most fruits and the richest known source is the fruit of the Amazonian camu camu tree (*Myricaria dubia*). Other good sources include acerola cherries, guavas, oranges, lemons, elderberries, mangoes and tangerines. Lack of this nutrient causes scurvy, which has symptoms of bleeding gums, large bleeds into the skin, swollen joints, heart failure and ultimately can result in death.

Vitamin E – This vitamin is a potent antioxidant and protects immune system cells from damage. Research suggests that it may be valuable in preventing or treating a wide range of diseases including acne, allergies, eczema, menstrual period pain, and menopausal symptoms. It is found most abundantly in vegetable oils, nuts and seeds. Avocados are a good source.

Minerals

Boron – This trace element is crucial to the metabolism of calcium and magnesium. It activates vitamin D that in turn stimulates the absorption of calcium. Boron also seems to potentiate the effects of oestrogen in maintaining the health of bones and so it is of use in the prevention and treatment of osteoporosis. It is present in many fruits but only if the soil in which they were grown was rich in boron. This is more likely to be the case with organically grown fruit.

Calcium – This well-known for its role in building strong bones but it is also essential for the control of muscle and nerve functions. Calcium needs to be taken alongside magnesium, ideally in a ratio of 2:1 (2 parts calcium to 1 part magnesium). Although dairy foods are rich in calcium they are relatively deficient in magnesium with a ratio of 11:1 for cow's milk and 22:1 for cheese.

A high-dairy diet can decrease magnesium levels to the point where symptoms of deficiency develop. Although vegetable sources tend to have a lower overall calcium content, they contain it in a form that is perfectly balanced with magnesium at 2:1. Good sources include carob flour, almonds, Brazil nuts, figs, olives, walnuts and prunes. Fruits such as apples also contain a little calcium.

Iron – Iron is vital for the production of haemoglobin, the compound that carries oxygen around the body. Deficiency causes anaemia and the symptoms of fatigue, weakness, breathing difficulties and dizziness. Sources include dried apricots (3.4mg of iron per 100g of apricots), almonds (4.7mg of iron per 100g of almonds) and cocoa powder (10.5mg of iron per 100g of cocoa powder).

Magnesium – Low levels of magnesium are associated with heart disease, high blood pressure, premenstrual syndrome, insomnia, fatigue, irritability and muscle cramps. Vegetable sources are the main providers of this nutrient. It is abundant in nuts, especially almonds, cashews and Brazil nuts.

Phosphorus – This mineral has numerous roles to play in the body, usually when combined with other chemicals in the form of phosphates, such as calcium phosphate. It is hard to become deficient in phosphorus since it is present in most types of food. It is present in fruits and nuts.

Potassium – This is also found in many different foods but fruits are a particularly good source. It is important for controlling the functions of cells – its exchange with sodium across cell membranes is one of the key processes that drive cellular activity.

The balance between potassium and sodium in the diet is very important. A low potassium, high sodium diet is associated with some cancers and heart diseases such as high blood pressure and strokes. On the other hand a low sodium, high potassium diet seems to lessen the risk of these diseases. The key is to cut down salt (sodium chloride) intake and increase potassium rich foods. The potassium-to-sodium ratio in the diet should be greater than 5:1 (at least 5 times more potassium than sodium). Average Western diets are often at the potentially harmful ratio of 1:2. Fruits have a naturally high potassium-to-sodium ratio, for example apples are 90:1; peaches and plums around 150:1 and oranges 260:1. To promote a healthy potassium-to-sodium ratio, don't add salt to food but increase your fruit consumption.

Zinc – This nutrient is of prime importance in enzyme processes, hormonal function (such as insulin, growth hormone and sex hormones) and immune system health. It is vital for the healing of wounds and optimal performance of the senses of smell, taste and vision. It is very important in men in preventing prostate disease. Zinc is present in good amounts in many nuts including pecans, Brazil nuts, almonds, walnuts and hazelnuts.

Trace Elements

Copper – Copper is involved in enzyme functions, including iron absorption and the development of collagen in connective tissues. It is found in nuts such as Brazil nuts, almonds, hazelnuts and walnuts.

Chromium – This is essential for the proper control of sugar in the blood and is provided by fruits and nuts.

Manganese – Essential in the control of enzymatic processes such as blood sugar control, thyroid function and energy production. It is found in nuts (pecans, Brazil nuts, almonds, walnuts) and many spices.

Selenium – Important in the prevention and treatment of cancer, depression and other psychiatric disorders, infertility, immune deficiency and heart disease, selenium is found in Brazil nuts and oranges.

Antioxidants

Several of the nutrients mentioned above are antioxidants – including beta-carotene, and vitamins C and E. Free radicals can damage important cell materials such as proteins and DNA leading to an increased risk of cancer. They also create lipid peroxides, products of fat metabolism, which can increase the build up of fats in the walls of arteries leading to heart disease. Regular eating of orange and yellow fruits such as oranges and lemons and vitamin E sources, such as nuts and avocados, can reduce the risk of developing these problems. Lemons are too sour to eat as a peeled fruit; it is best to squeeze them and drink the juice mixed with water or other fruit juices. The juice of one freshly squeezed lemon taken each day can have powerful effects in preventing disease.

Food preparation

A further, and perhaps surprising, benefit of trees in nutrition is the use of wood for making the chopping boards used in food preparation. Wood has natural antiseptic qualities from its oils and resins that prevent the build-up of the bacteria that cause food poisoning. Using a wooden preparation board is in fact far more hygienic and safer than using a plastic board – it also makes cooking more of a pleasurable experience.

How can I use it?

In terms of prevention we can work with the ideas of nutritional medicine by eating a healthy and delicious diet including tree medicines such as nuts, fruits and oils. Make up your own muesli, fruit salads and juices, salad dressings and other dishes incorporating tree ingredients.

What could be a more natural medicine than picking an apple from a tree and sitting down to enjoy its wonderful taste and aroma? The reality is that often, by the time our food reaches us, it isn't very fresh and has been reared with artificial fertilizers, sprayed with carcinogenic pesticides and it may even be genetically modified. It becomes very important to insist on carefully and responsibly grown certified organic food. Although the cost of organic food is often rather more in financial terms, we have to consider that, in environmental terms, conventionally grown foods, quite literally, cost the earth.

It is great to eat food that you have grown yourself, fresh as can be – if you want to do this but don't have a garden then try renting an allotment instead. If you don't have enough time for this, then consider joining together with other people in a similar situation and grow food between you in a community garden. In some areas people have knocked down the fences separating their individual small gardens to create one huge community garden – a great idea.

There are a huge number of books that look at particular diets and the variety can be confusing. Unfortunately, most cookbooks are written with scant attention paid to health considerations. Look out for cookbooks where the author states that they have aimed to balance taste with health. It is often useful to consult a professional nutritionist to help steer a path through the conflicting dietary messages we get from books, official sources and the media. When illness is threatened or established it is definitely valuable to consult a professional nutritionist. A first consultation will take about an hour and treatment will consist of nutritional advice and usually prescription of nutritional supplements for a limited period of time.

5

Weathering the Storm –
Medicinal Trees at Risk

IT IS BECOMING increasingly clear that life on Earth depends on maintaining a delicate balance of relationships between all the many species
on the planet. Preservation of the planet's biodiversity (its many species
of flora and fauna) is central to the survival of our own species. We depend
on each other.

Trees are a major part of the world's rich tapestry of life forms. Forests
are the most biologically varied ecosystems on Earth and many plants can
only grow in the company of trees, in the special environments that trees
create. No one knows for sure how many different types of tree there are but
it has been estimated that there could be around 100,000 distinct species. It
is calculated that 9% of all tree species living today are globally threatened
with extinction.

Some of the richest areas of biodiversity on the planet are the rainforests
and these contain tens of thousands of species. They cover only about 6%
of the Earth's landmass but contain perhaps 50% of all living species. The
Peruvian rainforest has an average of 300 tree species per hectare; by contrast the number of tree species for the whole of North America is just 700
with an average of about 20 tree species per hectare of temperate forest. In
1996 researchers in Brazil found that a one hectare plot in the Santa Teresa
area of the Atlantic rainforest contained 476 different tree species! The

Atlantic rainforest used to cover about 1.2 million square kilometres, now it is reduced to 2–5% of that original size. Nonetheless it is still estimated to contain around 20,000 different plant species.

The tropical rain forests are extraordinarily rich in species but temperate forests, though less diverse, are also immensely important; they are also facing severe threats. Deforestation is not as pronounced an issue in temperate forests; the overall size of most temperate woodland is stable or even increasing, although there are regional differences. The total forested area of Europe and North America is slowly increasing but in Asia it is significantly decreasing. The size of a forest, however, says nothing about its quality. We have lost many primary, or old growth, forests and gained new intensively managed forests. These latter are often 'tree monocultures', with a single species being planted, most often a conifer rather than a broadleaved tree. Such plantations are poor in biodiversity, giving little support to other plant, insect and animal species.

Temperate forest covers over 2 billion hectares of the planet's surface. Around 42% of the world's total temperate forest is in Russia, with North America accounting for 32%, Asia 10%, non-Russian Europe 8%, Australasia 5%, Latin America 2% and Africa 1%. A study by the European Commission and the United Nations Commission for Europe (published in October 2000) found that 36% of European trees were classed as being 'healthy' (they had no loss of leaves or needles), 41% were at the 'warning stage' (showing some signs of defoliation) and a worrying 20% were classed as 'damaged' (they had lost over 25% of their leaves or needles). The report found that while tree health had improved in 15% of the sites previously tested it had worsened in 30% of sites. There had been some improvements in western and central Europe but a worsening in the Mediterranean. The main reason for the poor health of European trees is damage from environmental pollution with atmospheric nitrogen and sulphur.

In Africa the threats to woodland include felling of forests for agriculture, overgrazing, forest fires, excessive logging, over-harvesting of fuel wood and military conflicts. Woodland in Africa covers 520 million hectares and it has the second largest area of tropical forest after South America. According to a report by the United Nations Food and Agriculture Organization in 2000, deforestation in Africa occurs at a rate that is over twice the world average and it lost over 10% of its total forest mass between 1980 and 1995. Constant political unrest throughout the continent has meant that a sustained programme of forest conservation management has been impossible.

Studies estimate that we will lose 20% of all the Earth's species (flora and fauna) within the next 25 years. Throughout the 1990s the rate of loss of tropical rainforests has been 1% a year. At this rate, by the end of the twenty-first century they will all have been destroyed. In the process man may also have altered the global environment to such an extent that human life on earth is no longer possible.

THE CAUSES OF TREE LOSS

There are many reasons why many forests and individual tree species are threatened with destruction. Often a combination of factors combine to cause the decline of a particular area of woodland or a particular species of tree.

Agriculture

Many areas of forest have been cleared for the purpose of growing crops or raising cattle. Crops are usually of one type only and replace the extensive biodiversity of natural woodland with 'deserts' of a single species. Forest soils are not always suited to crop growing and can quickly become depleted. When this occurs the growers move on to devastate another area of trees leaving a wasteland behind them. Cattle ranching is seldom of benefit to local people, most of the profits going to the owners of multinational burger chains. Here, forest destruction results in little more than supporting an industry peddling an unhealthy and unnecessary product.

Overgrazing, particularly by goats, results in trees being 'ring-barked' (an area of bark is removed from all around the trees' girth) which kills the trees. Another destructive aspect of agriculture is the use of fertilizers, pesticides and herbicides that alter the nature of the soil and poison water sources, and animal and plant life including trees themselves.

Expansion of settlements

As the world's population grows, more land is given over to housing and amenities. Expanding population centres result in the surrounding woodland being cut down, not only in the developing world but in the developed world as well.

Fires

Forest fires are a natural phenomenon and are sometimes an essential part of the life cycle of a forest. However, if fires occur too frequently or too extensively they can cause massive damage. More widespread human invasion of forests increases the risk of accidental fire. There are also indications that global warming is causing fires to become more numerous and more severe due to woodlands being drier and easier to ignite. As forests become more fragmented they are more susceptible to the damaging effects of fire.

Invasive plants

The introduction of non-indigenous plants into woodlands can prove disastrous as they compete with more useful indigenous species. Forests' ecosystems operate delicate balances between all of their constituent species; the introduction of an invasive plant can have devastating effects.

Political disturbance

Political instability may mean that woodland conservation is not seen as a priority and the fate of trees is neglected. Where a nation is in a constant state of political flux huge problems can develop over many years.

Local use

Excessive local harvesting of woodland products, such as wood for fuel, can decimate forests. Even when only fallen wood is harvested it can have significant repercussions if harvested too extensively. This is because woodlands need fallen trees to be broken down by weather, fungi and insects so that they can return their stored nutrition to the soil so that other trees and plants can thrive.

Mining and exploration

Large tracts of trees are felled to accommodate mining developments, quarries, and in exploration and surveys for natural resources.

Tourism and leisure

Forests' ecosystems have been disrupted by insensitive recreational developments and excessive human presence.

Pollution

Pollution with sulphur dioxide, nitrogen oxides and ozone has lead to a total of 61% of European trees showing signs of damage, and similar pollution affects trees globally. So-called 'acid rain' is produced by toxic emissions from road vehicles, industrial plants and electricity generating centres. The effects of pollution by agricultural chemicals are equally devastating.

Over-exploitation of forest products

Certain species are under threat of extinction after being over-harvested to satisfy demand for their use in such products as medicines, foods and other commercial materials. Research shows that excessive harvesting of trees for use as medicines is a major reason for at least 200 tree species being classed as being at risk.

Logging

Logging by the timber trade has resulted in truly appalling levels of deforestation, especially in tropical regions. Aggressive large-scale logging produces devastation, not just by the logging itself. Huge roads are needed to allow the loggers into the forest and then extract the timber out. These roads slice the forest up into smaller and smaller patches making it easier for them to be encroached upon. As the companies move on, they frequently leave displaced and abandoned workers behind them. These people are often given little alternative but to devastate more forest in order to try and raise crops upon which to survive.

All of the above issues can lead to destruction of tree habitats and the diminishing or loss of specific tree species. But what exactly are the consequences of these actions?

THE CONSEQUENCES OF TREE LOSS

Global warming

Forests act as 'sinks' for the main greenhouse gas, carbon dioxide. This means that they absorb carbon dioxide naturally as part of the process of photosynthesis. The absorbed carbon is stored in the wood of the trees. With a reduction in the number of trees to control carbon dioxide, the levels of this gas will continue to rise leading to world temperature change. Climate change may lead to an increase in dramatic weather conditions with floods, droughts and extreme winds causing immense damage and disruption.

Soil erosion

Forest cover reduces soil erosion. Exposing tracts of land to the open air without tree cover or substantial hedging allows wind and water to remove topsoil thus impairing both the stability and fertility of the land. Roots knit the soil together and prevent landslides. Trees serve an important purpose alongside inland waterways, rail and road systems to maintain the integrity of banks and prevent disasters.

Species loss

Destruction of woodland habitat also destroys the habitats of many species and this can lead to their decline or even extinction. At risk are lichens, mosses, flowering plants, insects and animals. Palaeontologists believe that climate change caused some of the great extinctions of the past.

Loss of native peoples

There are many groups of indigenous peoples who have built their homes and established their culture in woodland environments. By taking the trees away we put these cultures at risk and destroy their unique qualities and achievements.

Spread of disease

Disruptions in the balance of nature can lead to an increase in illnesses. In woodland, the balance between species can be altered with species that cause or carry disease increasing in numbers. The rise in temperatures resulting from global warming may promote the spread of tropical diseases. Depletion of the ozone layer puts people at higher risk of skin cancer.

Loss of recreational areas

Forests are widely used as places for exploration, walking, and contemplation. Without them our health-giving and recreational resources become severely reduced.

Loss of resources

As trees disappear, so do the products they produce. Trees not only provide us with building materials, fuel and paper but forests also yield gums, mushrooms, honey, perfumes, materials for crafts, fibres, dyes, fodder and many other materials in addition to foods and medicines.

Loss of foods

Valuable tree foods both for us and for wildlife are under threat. We depend on tree fruits for much of the healthier part of our diets and the vital role that certain nutrients play in keeping us well is at last being understood. We could lose trees that are already established as of major nutritional significance such as the Brazil nut tree (source of selenium) and less well-known trees that have huge health-promoting potential such as the camu camu tree (*Myricaria dubia*) that is the richest known source of vitamin C.

Loss of medicines

Some trees are directly threatened because we know that they have medicinal properties and they are being harvested to death. We may also be losing trees whose therapeutic activities we are not yet aware of. Important medicines could be disappearing without us knowing what we have lost. Research programmes are identifying chemicals that offer hope in the treatment of severe diseases such as human immunodeficiency virus (HIV) infections and AIDS. Forests are natural pharmacies – we cannot afford to lose the remedies they contain.

Loss of knowledge of medicines and conservation

We are not only losing medicinal plants themselves, we are also losing traditional knowledge about their use. Destruction of plant habitats is destroying the homes of indigenous peoples and consequently of their culture, lifestyle and ancestral knowledge, including medical knowledge. But not only this, tribal peoples also have extensive understanding of plant conservation and can help show us how to conserve and create tree habitats.

The Mebengokre ('People of the Waters' Source') tribe in Brazil have long been expert at developing and maintaining their own ecosystem. They plant forest islands (apete) of useful plants to increase areas of beneficial biodiversity. Heaps of manure from termite and ant nests are placed in moisture-retaining depressions in the ground. These fertile areas are then planted with medicinal and edible trees and herbs at the start of the rainy season. These islands have varied regions of light, shade, temperature and moisture providing a selection of microclimates to meet the differing needs of many plants. They provide sources of remedies and foods, and support other animal and insect life. The Mebengokre have an understanding of plants that grow well together, and talk of them as being 'good neighbours'. Such 'companion planting' can improve plants' overall health, growth rates and disease resistance.

Loss of our humanity

When trees disappear physically, do we all lose spiritually? The story of life on Earth is the story of the interaction between animals, plants, land and water. As the dominant animals on the planet, we have a duty of care to all other organisms with which we share the planet. If we are willing to let other species disappear out of apathy, ignorance or lifestyle choices, what does that say about us? If we lose our places of sanctuary and contemplation, our natural sources of inspiration, we may find ourselves equally spiritually bereft.

TREES AT RISK

Conservation of existing forests and the creation of new ones is one of the main strategies to reverse the ecological decline. Before considering the solutions to the global problem of deforestation lets look at which medicinal trees are actually considered to be at risk.

The IUCN (The World Conservation Union) is the main organization involved in collecting and publishing details of the world's endangered plant species. They list five main categories to describe to what extent a plant is at risk of decreasing in numbers or even disappearing entirely. These are as follows:

Vulnerable – These trees face a high risk of extinction in the wild in the medium-term future;

Endangered – Trees in this group face a very high risk of extinction in the wild in the near future;

Critically endangered – The trees in this category are a cause for major concern since they face an extremely high risk of extinction in the wild in the immediate future;

Extinct in the wild – These trees no longer appear in their normal habitats and only exist in cultivation or in small, protected areas of preservation;

Extinct – These are trees that we have lost – they can no longer be found anywhere on the planet, either in the wild or in cultivation.

In addition to these, there is a lower risk category in which tree species of concern are placed and then monitored to ensure that they don't become more threatened.

The danger is greatest for trees whose roots, wood or bark are used as medicines. It is much easier to harvest leaves, flowers, fruits and seeds in a sustainable fashion. The removal of roots means threatening the health of the whole tree. When wood is harvested, the whole tree tends to be cut down or large branches are successively lopped off until the tree dies. Only small patches of bark can be removed from trees without destroying the water and nutrient transport system of the tree and thereby killing it.

Of the medicinal trees mentioned in this book at least 26 are causing concern that they are threatened with becoming extinct in the wild. These include:

Aquilaria malaccensis (Agarwood)

Betholletia excelsa (Brazil nut)

Boswellia sacra (Frankincense)

Cedrus libani var libani (Cedar of Lebanon)

Commiphora wightii (Guggul)

Cupressus sempervirens (Italian cypress)

Garcinia kola (Garcinia)

Ginkgo biloba (Maidenhair tree)

Guaiacum coulteri (Guaiacum)

Guaiacum officinale (Lignum vitae)

Guaiacum sanctum (Guaiacum)

Guarea macrophylla (Guarea)

Ilex paraguaiensis (Yerba maté)

Liquidambar orientalis var integriloba (Storax)

Liquidambar orientalis var orientalis (Storax)

Magnolia officinalis (Magnolia)

Magnolia sinensis (Magnolia)

Magnolia wilsonii (Magnolia)

Prunus africana (Red stinkwood)

Pterocarpus marsupium (Malabar kino)

Pterocarpus santalinus (Red sandalwood)

Santalum album (Sandalwood)

Tabebuia species (Pau d'arco)

Taxus brevifolia (Pacific yew)

Taxus wallichiana (Himalayan yew)

Warburgia salutaris (Pepper-bark tree)

This list covers many of the important medicinal trees at risk but several other healing trees not referred to in this book are also in danger. A recent study of medicinal trees in Ecuador found that several species are simply vanishing due to unsustainable collection for use as remedies. These trees include holy wood (*Bursera graveolens*) that is used as a pain-reliever, and a type of walnut (*Juglans neotropica*).

While some of the trees listed as at risk in the wild are widespread in cultivation (such as *Ginkgo biloba*), others are very hard to cultivate because they have specific habitat requirements such as soil type, temperature, shade, and dependency on other species of plants and insects. Some can be cultivated but are so slow growing that it is difficult to create a viable dynamic population. Although it is reassuring that many trees can survive in cultivation this can never be a direct replacement for the wild state. In the wild trees have complex and mutually supportive relationships with other species of flora and fauna that are difficult to recreate in a controlled habitat. Loss of trees from an area in the wild also affects the character and special meaning of a place; we lose an aspect of the 'personality' of the region concerned.

Specific examples of medicinal trees that are under threat include:

Red Stinkwood

One of the medicinal trees causing most serious concern at present is the African tree, Red stinkwood (*Prunus africana* or *Pygeum africana*). It grows in mountainous areas and owes its name to the fact that its bark, leaves and fruit have the potent smell of bitter almonds.

In traditional African medicine Red stinkwood has been used to treat chest pain, fevers and stomachache but it has become in great demand in the West for the benefits it brings in the common male disease, benign prostatic hyperplasia. Research has confirmed the effectiveness of *Prunus africana* bark in treating this unpleasant condition and demand for natural treatments for prostate disease is so high that populations of this tree have been decimated. It is calculated that the European and American market for *Prunus africana* in 2000 was US$220 million, with around 3,500 tonnes of bark currently being harvested each year, principally in Cameroon. Unsustainable harvesting has led to it being placed on the CITES (Convention on International Trade in Endangered Species) Appendix II list of threatened plants which allows a controlled trade in sustainably harvested bark. It is also now growing in protected environments in several areas.

Although *Prunus africana is* a slow-growing tree, populations are said to regenerate well when given the opportunity to do so by preventing their exploitation. However, because of the high prices this tree commands, there is a large trade in poaching the medicinal bark. In an encouraging move, the International Center for Research in Agroforestry (ICRAF) is assisting farmers to cultivate this tree and is training them in sustainable harvesting techniques so that they can earn a reasonable living. An 'ecolabel' certification scheme is being developed to prove that *Prunus africana* bark has been ethically produced.

Sandalwood

Sandalwood (*santalum album*) has one of the most entrancing scents of all woods. The distilled volatile oil is extensively used for incense, perfumes and as a medicine. It is used in aromatherapy for urinary infections, as a sexual tonic and to help relieve stress and tension states. In India the tree is seen as being sacred, its oil having spiritual significance, and sandalwood incense is used as part of religious ceremonies. It is thought to have originated in Indonesia and then spread to India. It also grows in China, the Philippines and Australia.

The Sandalwood tree is now at risk in many areas due to overexploitation. It is hard to harvest this tree in a sustainable manner because the heartwood (the wood at the centre of the trunk) is used in medicine; in order to obtain it the whole tree is cut down or uprooted. It takes between 30–50 years for trees to grow to a stage where they produce sufficient heartwood.

This means that replacement of natural stocks is very slow. This tree is also threatened by its use in the timber trade, by a particular tree disease (especially in India), by forest fires and by destruction of its habitat for agriculture and cattle grazing. In India, trade in sandalwood is restricted but there is also a large problem with smuggling. Australia is the main source of sandalwood chips that are used in manufacturing incense. The tree is classed as being vulnerable except in India, where sandalwood problems may be worsening, it is classed at a lower level of risk. There is little financial incentive to cultivate this tree because of the length of time it takes to harvest the heartwood. Nonetheless some efforts are being made to regenerate stocks and a project in Indonesia has been launched with the aim of growing 30,000 hectares of sandalwood forest over 15 years.

SAVING OUR TREES

The situation regarding endangered trees is ever changing, with new developments constantly occurring and new information coming to light. Some non-medicinal trees are harvested for medicines because they are mistaken for a true medicinal species. More sinisterly, they might be collected in order to be passed off knowingly as the real thing. The incentives to mislead customers in this way are large because the value of medicinal plants, like all other commodities, rises as supply decreases.

One of the purposes of this book is to raise awareness of tree medicines to add to the many other good reasons to conserve trees. Although we are right to be worried about the future of life on Earth if we continue to destroy our forests at the current rate, this doesn't mean that we are unable to do anything about it. It is not too late to redress the balance; we have not gone too far just yet. So what can we do to make a difference?

The factors involved in deforestation are several and complex, so it is not surprising that is are a large number of ways we can contribute towards a solution. These can be achieved at the level of the individual; the group; nationally, and internationally. Although the actions that each one of us can take may seem small in the face of the size of the problem, if enough people take the same actions independently of each other then the effects can add up to have a huge positive influence. Bear in mind that there is an overlap between the levels of action and as individuals we can contribute towards the work of groups, who can influence the policies of nations, who can come together to act collectively towards a common purpose.

Individual Action

We can begin to have less impact on the planet's resources and help to ease the pressure on trees by carrying out a 'lifestyle audit'. This means that we examine the way we live our lives to see if there are any areas that we can make small yet significant changes that will help ease the burden that the planet has to bear. This includes reflecting on how we spend our money and our time in our daily lives. Areas to think about, and additional things we can do, include:

- **travel** – one of the major causes of global warming is emission of greenhouse gases from burning fossil fuels in motor vehicles. By altering our lifestyles to reduce these emissions we can contribute towards lowering the pollution to a level that trees can cope with better. Think about how often you use your car. Avoid using it for short journeys when you could easily walk or cycle. This will help the planet and improve your health. Make a deal with yourself that you'll walk or cycle in good weather and only use the car if the weather is too severe. Could you use public transport more? It solves parking problems and is often quicker.

- **energy use** – the other significant greenhouse gas creator from the burning of fossil fuels is the electricity generating industry. Try and be electricity conscious, turn off lights, heating and appliances when you are not using them. Use energy saving devices and consider the possibility of meeting some of your own energy requirements by installing solar or wind power generators.

- **become 'carbon neutral'** – even if we cut our energy requirements to a minimum we will still be directly responsible for generating waste emissions by using transport, electricity and consumer products. It is estimated that the average household uses up 2 tonnes of carbon a year in heating and light. We can offset this by planting trees that will absorb carbon dioxide to compensate for the amount of carbon dioxide we create. You can do this by planting trees in your garden – if you have enough space – or by sponsoring tree plantings by tree charities. One way of doing this is by donating to 'Tree Aid' (*see* Resources) who will plant trees in Africa on your behalf to counter global warming and also to provide much-needed food and soil stabilization for local communities.
  An organization called 'Future Forests' (*see* Resources) in the UK will work out your annual carbon dioxide production for you and advise you on how many trees you need to plant to neutralize it. In Australia an

initiative called Greenfleet provides an opportunity for motorists to offset the carbon dioxide produced by their cars by planting trees on their behalf. Similar organizations are beginning to appear in other countries.

- **forest gardening** – in our gardens we can remember that trees provide food, shade and beauty just as well as other plants. If you have space, try and incorporate trees into your garden design. If you are lucky enough to have a lot of space why not plant an orchard? An area of fruit trees is a joyous thing; you can provide a large supply of fruits, attract beneficial insects and create an area of peace to sit in the shade on a summer afternoon. Children love orchards and delight in eating fruit that they've picked themselves.

  A system of interplanting medicinal and edible trees with vegetables in a complementary way is known as 'forest gardening' (*see* Robert A De J. Hart's *Forest Gardening*, in the Bibliography). If you don't have a garden try renting an allotment.

- **repair, reuse and recycle** – we can conserve Earth's resources, including wood products, by trying to replace the products we use less often. When an item is broken, have it repaired rather than throwing it away and buying another one. Try to reuse things. For instance, if you no longer need or want an item of furniture pass it on to someone who does. This can often be done via a local authority or charity.

- **be an ethical consumer** – one of the major threats to trees, particularly rainforest trees, is the timber industry. Indiscriminate logging has devastated the world's woodland resources. Avoid buying wooden products made from threatened tree species; if the supplier cannot guarantee that the wood comes from a sustainable source, don't buy it. Use caution when buying everything from furniture and window frames to ornaments and toilet seats.

  Buying guaranteed sustainably harvested and fairly traded rainforest products is a good way of helping indigenous peoples to derive a low impact income from the rainforest and help to conserve it. Also, we can all choose to boycott fast-food burger outlets that fell forests to make way for their cattle to graze.

- **buy locally** – support your local craft workers by buying their products. Bear in mind that you can commission items such as pieces of furniture from local experts. This helps to keep traditional skills alive and is often no more expensive than buying a good-quality piece off the shelf. If you buy work made from local materials you will also encourage traditional woodland management in your area and have an item that is more than just an object but that also connects you with your community and locale.

Group Action

Much of the individual action above can be extended to groups. A number of you could join together with others to start a community garden. Land can be bought, or rented (perhaps from a local authority), and a forest garden established and maintained by several people, spreading the load and increasing the yields – in terms of food, and also in terms of friendship and meaningful social interaction. Other forms of group action to save trees and support the benefits of trees include:

- **shared transport** – vehicle sharing schemes offer a system where people can share car journeys. This system is particularly useful for sharing transport to and from work.

- **lobby groups** – organizations such as Greenpeace and Friends of the Earth actively campaign to stop environmental destruction and influence individuals and governments to protect the planet (*see* Resources for these and other related organizations). By joining such groups and supporting them both financially and by participating in campaigns you can make a real difference.

- **conservation groups** – organizations such as the National Trust and the Woodland Trust in the UK and the Land Trust Alliance in the USA buy and conserve land, protecting its biodiversity for ourselves and future generations. We can support their vital work by becoming members; this will also often give us access to areas of outstanding natural beauty owned by the group. Taking our children to visit such places can engender a love of nature in them and inspire them to care for them as they grow older.

- **non-governmental organizations** – initiatives such as the Global Trees Campaign (*see* Resources) provide high-quality information on the status of the world's tree resources and campaign for tree conservation and develop projects to save endangered species.

- **botanic gardens** – scientific botanic gardens such as those at Edinburgh and Chelsea and their counterparts around the world, such as the National Tropical Botanical Gardens in Florida and Hawaii, grow many endangered species within their grounds. They also conduct much research and educational work.

Several gardens, such as the Australian National Botanic Gardens, act as centres for conserving their country's indigenous plants. Kew Gardens has launched the Millennium Seed Bank project which has been described by the naturalist Sir David Attenborough as 'perhaps the most significant conservation initiative ever undertaken'. The scheme aims to collect and conserve the seeds of 10% (over 24,000) of the world's seed-bearing plants and 100% of UK seed-bearing plants.

- **responsible businesses** – increasingly, companies are attempting to present themselves as being 'environmentally friendly'. While this can often amount to superficial window dressing, there are real opportunities for environmental benefits. By reducing the production of greenhouse gases, by reducing energy needs and subsidizing staff to use public transport, each company can make a difference. It is also possible for businesses to become 'carbon neutral' by auditing how many trees they need to plant to offset their annual carbon dioxide production. Companies already working with Future Forests in this way include Whole Earth Foods, Mazda Cars UK Ltd and the advertising agency J Walter Thompson.

National Action

Individuals and organizations can influence governments to enact policies and laws that protect trees and the environment. Government initiatives can include:

- **restrict greenhouse gas emissions** – it is incumbent upon all national governments to do all they can to reduce fossil fuel pollution of the atmosphere. This can be achieved by making public transport more attractive than private car use, investing in alternative energy production systems and imposing restrictions on business pollution.

- **educating the public** – in the UK in 2000 we witnessed companies obtaining significant public support for reductions in fuel prices while, at the same time, the nation was suffering from its worst floods on record – a direct result of global warming caused by excessive fossil fuel usage! Governments need to explain why fuel costs must continue to be high in order to inhibit indiscriminate use.

- **conserve old forests and create new ones** – it is important that old forests are conserved as they have a greater biodiversity and absorb more carbon dioxide than new forests. We also need to plant the right kind of trees for the area concerned – fast-growing conifer forests do not have the same qualities as slower-growing broad leaf forests. While we must focus on the rainforests we also need to remember that less extensive and well-known forests also need to be conserved or regenerated (such as the highland forests of Scotland – see Carifran Wildwood in Resources).

- **Make funds available** – to invest in tree conservation and new plantations. Also to subsidize companies which invest in long-term strategies to cultivate endangered slow-growing trees for medicinal use.

- **Encourage and support businesses** – that operate in a sustainable and ethical manner and legislate against those that don't.

- **Encourage small timber businesses** – localized timber companies have more incentive to nurture their resources than huge timber conglomerates that can afford to strip out an area and then move on leaving devastation behind them.

- **Put woodlands at the centre of the community** – governments need to show that they value trees by having strict preservation and regeneration policies and resisting developments that harm them.

- **Ensure intellectual property rights** – for medicinal knowledge are acknowledged and rewarded and that profits are kept within the communities that generate them. When a pharmaceutical company discovers a new drug with the help of an indigenous healer, the whole community involved should be properly rewarded and all monies should benefit the whole community.

International Action

Much national action can be extended by international agreements, thereby increasing their scope and impact. International treaties can have a huge influence, but only if they are fully complied with and enforced. International actions can include:

- **Cut national debts** – many countries are allowing truly horrific logging programmes to proceed in order to meet bills for international debts. It is imperative that such debts are cancelled by the wealthy Western nations.

- **Impose trade embargoes** – nations can agree to observe worldwide action to restrict or outlaw trade in endangered species defined by groups such as CITES. Species under Appendix I of CITES are banned from international trade, those under Appendix II are controlled.

- **Set global environmental goals** – governments can meet to establish targets for environmental aims such as the Kyoto Protocol on climate change set in 1997. This aims to reduce carbon dioxide emissions across the planet by 2010. Having set targets and made agreements, all participating countries need to abide by the spirit of them as well as by the letter!

- **Limit the environmental impact of new technologies** – all new technologies must be developed with safety as a primary aim. For instance, there is an urgent need to set internationally agreed protocols for coping with the challenges of genetic engineering which otherwise has the potential to wreak enormous havoc with the delicate and complex balance of nature.

- **Establish ways in which population growth can be limited** – a hugely expanding human population has to be accommodated somehow and the pressure to destroy forests in order to provide settlements is strong. We must recognize that the Earth is only so large and find ways of ensuring that we do not outgrow our home.

From all of this the resounding message is that we can do something about the current perilous situation – both as individuals and as groups. When Bill Mollison, the Tasmanian originator of the ecological farming concept called 'Permaculture' (for permanent agriculture), was asked if the planet could be saved from environmental disaster, his reply was – 'Will plants grow?'

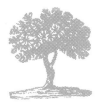

6

Bearing Fruit –
The Future of Tree Medicine

IN PART 2 OF THIS book, you will find profiles of trees that are helpful for treating the many minor problems including headaches, indigestion, flatulence, anxiety, sleeplessness, coughs and colds. You will also find trees that can make a contribution towards relieving serious disease such as diabetes and cancer. There may be some uses that surprise you, such as providing contraceptives for family planning. Trees are so wide-ranging in their scope as medicines and so versatile that we might wonder why the word 'treatment' isn't spelt 'treetment'! Trees then are a major part of the healing tradition. But what does the future hold for tree medicine?

As we have seen, the first thing that needs to be done to ensure the future of tree medicine is to protect the future of the trees from which they are derived. But it is not sufficient just to halt the destruction; it is also necessary to plant new forests to regenerate what we have already lost.

In New Zealand, an initiative called 'Project Crimson' has been set up to protect two of the country's most endangered trees. These are the crimson flowered rata and pohutukawa trees (*Metrosideros* species) that are classed as 'iron-hearted myrtles' due to the deep red colour of their heartwood. Between 1990 and 2000 volunteers working for the project have planted a remarkable 200,000 trees. Also in New Zealand, the government has announced that it will make it illegal to conduct logging of any publicly owned forests from March 2002. While it would be better to stop the logging right now, this is nonetheless a huge step forward.

TREES IN PUBLIC PLACES

Another good reason for more widespread planting of trees is as an element in what might be termed 'environmental medicine'. Trees offer valuable shade that can help to prevent direct contact with sunlight, so reducing the risk of developing skin cancer. In the future, we may see more open public spaces planted with trees for this purpose. We need to have the option to choose shade in our public places. Many streets, car parks, civic plazas, and entertainment and arts complexes are completely devoid of outside cover. Children and animals are particularly prone to developing dehydration in intense heat. This is a particular problem in large unshaded car parks where prolonged exposure to sunlight in hot cars poses a significant risk. Trees provide the ideal 'breathable' shade with cooled air and dappled light filtering through the leaves.

Widespread tree planting also helps to keep the air clean, so preventing and easing chest conditions such as asthma. In addition, trees engender positive thoughts and feelings, *and* they help us to feel relaxed and more purposeful. Perhaps in the future we will appreciate the value of trees in relieving psychiatric disease such as anxiety and alienation, especially in inner cities. Tree planting should become a more prominent feature of city planning and regeneration because of its ability to promote the health of inhabitants and visitors alike.

CULTIVATING TREE MEDICINES

Medicinal trees need to be cultivated more extensively for commercial harvesting of tree products in order to protect wild stocks. Cultivation of trees for medicines has the potential to provide a reasonable income for indigenous farmers, especially in impoverished areas such as parts of South America and Africa. At the moment this needs to take place alongside the sustainable harvesting of wild trees, but eventually, as cultivation becomes more widespread, the vast majority of tree medicines should be harvested from cultivated sources rather than wild. Most trees can be cultivated and many can be coppiced.

Coppicing is the craft of cutting back trees so that they produce several rapidly-growing bush-like stems. Coppiced trees can be harvested on a regular basis every few years after which the stems regenerate. This practice allows you to obtain a higher yield per planted area, growth is quicker so you can harvest earlier, and it is easier to gather the tree products since the coppiced trees are lower and easier to get at. Most importantly the required products can be harvested from the tree without harming it. In fact, properly coppiced trees live longer than trees left to grow naturally. This method can be used for gathering all tree parts but it is especially good for taking bark and wood as you cannot take much of these from a mature tree without severely limiting its chances of survival.

Ethnobotany

Of prime importance for the future of tree medicine is the continuing development of a new science called ethnobotany. The term 'ethnobotany' was coined by American botanist John W Harshberger in 1895. It derives from 'ethno' – the study of people, and 'botany' – the study of plants. Ethnobotanists are scientists who look at the relationship between people and plants. Their study covers all the ways that people interact with plants, from using them as foods to making shelters, boats, tools, and even the making and use of plant dyes. One of the major areas for their research is the use of plants as medicines. As part of their studies, ethnobotanists will live for periods of time with indigenous peoples to record and understand their traditional knowledge of plant uses. Much ethnobotanical work has been carried out in areas where indigenous tribes still live their lives in touch with their ancestral origins such as in South America and Africa.

It is being increasingly appreciated that, even in Western developed societies, there is much traditional plant knowledge still existing in the memories of the elder members of our communities that needs to be discovered and recorded before it is lost. In England, Gabrielle Hatfield (*see* Bibliography) has studied the ethnobotany of East Anglia and a project called 'Ethnomedica' (*see* Resources) has been launched to gather information about the traditional use of healing plants throughout the UK. In North America Daniel E Moerman has compiled a remarkable compendium about the use of plants by Native Americans, especially as medicines, in his book *Native American Ethnobotany*.

Ethnobotanists have gathered much fascinating material on the way we use plants to aid our health. One example is the way that some African tribes use trees to protect them against the potentially harmful effects of their diet. The Masai people live mainly on a diet of milk, meat and blood from their cattle. They have, in theory, one of the worst diets imaginable. It is particularly high in cholesterol, far higher than even the worst Western diets. Yet the Masai have healthy cholesterol levels. How come? The answer seems to lie in their use of tree barks in cooking. They add the bark of trees such as acacia (*Acacia goetzei* and *Albizzia anthelmintica*) to the pot when they cook meat. Studies have shown that these tree barks are effective in lowering cholesterol levels.

In recognition of the tremendous value of traditional plant knowledge the National Botanical Institute of South Africa has established a database called 'Medbase' which contains details of 300 of South Africa's most important medicinal plants. The database includes information on distribution, cultivation and conservation issues concerning each plant as well as ethnobotanical data about medicinal uses. The primary objective of the initiative is to encourage responsible land use in the country in order to conserve native herbal remedies and exploit them in a sustainable manner. The aim is to protect the trees, and use their products to improve the health and wealth of indigenous peoples.

One of the prime potential outcomes for ethnobotanical research is the identification of plants that can act as the starting point for the development of new drugs. Consequently, several pharmaceutical companies and special interest groups have funded ethnobotanical studies. When new medicine is developed in this way, a question then arises about ownership of the information that led to the medicine's discovery. In the past it has been all too common that the contribution of the people who have been the guardians of healing wisdom – the traditional physicians – has not been acknowledged. The situation is improving with the recognition of intellectual property rights and an increasing tendency to reward individuals and, more importantly, whole communities. It is vital for the future of tree medicines that this happens as it is another means by which rainforests and other woodlands can survive, giving their inhabitants an income and providing others with a disincentive to ruin their environment.

TRADITIONAL HEALING

Ethnobotany provides a link between the past and the future of plant medicines, and ethnobotanists have an essential role to play in preserving the traditional knowledge of healers. But, what of the traditional healers themselves and their practice of natural medicine? Many healers have now been displaced by the spread of Western medicine but traditional healers can still be found in many areas including South America and Africa.

The World Health Organisation encourages the preservation of natural healing wisdom and promotes its integration with Western healthcare. It is crucial for communities worldwide and for the plants they use, that traditional and conventional practitioners are given equal respect and that they work closely alongside each other. Orthodox medicine is, by and large, excellent at treating and managing medical emergencies such as those requiring surgical procedures. It is also tremendously helpful in chronic disorders. However, many drugs offer more problems than benefits and there is a lack of safe and effective treatment for many chronic conditions such as eczema and viral infections like the common cold. This is where the natural healer can help, by giving remedies that are, on the whole, gentler and safer and by helping successfully with chronic problems.

Another benefit of plant medicines is that they provide remedies that can strengthen and support the body's natural functions in a positive dynamic way. Plants that have these qualities are often described as 'tonics'. Tree tonics include immune boosters like elderflower and berries, digestive tonics such as quassia (*Picrasma excelsa*) and trees that strengthen the nervous system such as Jamaica dogwood (*Piscidia erythrina*).

One of the essential arts of the herbalist is to combine individual herbs so that they work together synergistically – that is to say, that the blended herbs work together more effectively than would any of the herbs given on their own. In China in particular a number of ancient mixtures are so well established that they have become famous formulations that are widely prescribed. Western herbalists rarely use ready-made formulas but instead blend by hand a mix of individual herbs for each patient, tending to prescribe around five herbs in any given mixture. When conventional doctors give herbs they tend to just give one at a time, this can mean that the success of the treatment is more limited.

EDUCATION AND LEGISLATION

The UK is unique in having several universities that offer courses in herbal medicine. These courses last 3–5 years and cover all the basic medical sciences (such as anatomy and physiology) as well as core traditional medicine elements such as botany, philosophy and herbal materia medica. Herbal practitioners so trained belong to a professional body with a complaints and disciplinary procedure and carry appropriate insurance for their activities. They also have to take part in compulsory continuing professional development in order to keep their knowledge up to date. All these factors help to protect the public and let people know that they are in safe and well-trained hands. The future of plant medicine as a proper and full discipline of medicine depends on courses such as these developing in other countries. The herbal profession is very small in countries such as the USA where legislation varies between states and the practice of herbalism is often prohibited.

There is a need for pharmacists to be better trained in the use of over-the-counter plant remedies so that everyone is able to visit their local chemist and receive sound advice about which preparation is most suitable for a given condition. This is even more important in health food shops where staff tend to have very little training in the remedies they stock and about medical conditions in general.

Even in the UK herbal practitioners find themselves in a precarious position. At present they have no properly defined legal status and it is possible for anyone to call themselves a medical herbalist. For tree medicines and other plant medicines to flourish in the future we need better legislation to regulate the activities of practitioners.

In the UK, the European Herbal Practitioners Association (EHPA) was formed in order to improve the legal status of herbalists and to protect the public right of access to safe and effective plant medicines, prescribed by competent and knowledgeable practitioners. The EHPA is working towards what is known as 'statutory self-regulation' of herbal practitioners and this will mean that only properly qualified and regulated herbalists will be able to offer their services to the public. This legislation will then provide a model for other European countries (and indeed countries worldwide) to adopt as a framework for the proper practice of plant medicine.

Legislative changes of this sort will make it possible for practitioners of plant medicines to be more fully integrated into the mainstream healthcare system. Already in the UK there are several herbalists working within doctor's surgeries, offering their services alongside conventional medical services. With proper legislation this situation can grow to the point where, in the future, it will be no more remarkable to consult a herbalist and receive a tree medicine, than it is now to consult a conventional doctor to be prescribed a tree-derived drug such as aspirin.

Future Research

Research has already revealed the capacity of many trees to improve our health and well-being but there is much more to come. One of the most fascinating areas is the potential of plant volatile oils to act as antibiotics. The main problem with many conventional antibiotics is that the infectious organisms they seek to destroy are rapidly becoming resistant to them. With repeated exposure to the same antibiotics bacteria evolve to adapt to the antibiotics, eventually rendering them useless. Such antibiotic-resistant micro-organisms have become known as 'superbugs'; they are portrayed as running riot unchecked by any conventional drugs. Such bacteria pose one of the most serious threats to our health in the years to come. Already there is a strain of bacterium called methycillin resistant *Staphylococcus aureus* (or MRSA) that is causing huge problems in hospitals. The mycobacterium that causes tuberculosis is also becoming antibiotic resistant and this is one of the reasons that there has been an increase in the incidence of TB over recent years. Part of the solution to this may be plant volatile oils.

Volatile oils

Volatile (essential) oils are the organic chemicals that make plants smell. When you smell camphor, or cloves or cinnamon, you are smelling the tree's volatile oil. All volatile oils have some antiseptic qualities to varying degrees. They are potently antibacterial and antifungal and some, such as the Madagascan tree ravensara (*Ravensara aromatica*) have antiviral properties.

Tea tree oil (*Melaleuca alternifolia*) is a broad spectrum antibacterial (against various bacteria including *Staphylococcus aureus* and *Pseudomonas aeruginosa*), antifungal (against *Candida albicans*, which causes thrush) and antiprotozoan (against *Trichomonas vaginalis*, a cause of vaginal infection). A close relative of tea tree called niaouli (*Melaleuca quinquinervia* or *viridiflora*) is antiviral against the herpes virus that causes cold sores. Other antibacterial tree volatile oils include cinnamon, cloves, pine and fir (*Abies* species).

Neem

For one final example of the health benefits that trees can bring, there is the case of the truly amazing neem tree. Neem (*Azadirachta indica*) is native to

India and Burma but has been introduced to many other countries in Africa, South America and the Caribbean. It has been of importance in Ayurvedic and Unani medicine in India for many centuries. It was given for a whole host of problems including malaria, fevers, loss of appetite, skin diseases, ulcers, rheumatism, leprosy, worm infestations – the list goes on. All parts of the tree have uses. As well as providing medicines, neem provides materials to make soap, toothpaste and skin lotions. Its wood is like mahogany and has been used as a substitute for that tree. It is a good fuel source and its leaves are used to feed animals. It is widely planted to provide shade.

Neem has one further trick up its sleeve that has proven of immense interest to researchers – it is an extraordinary insecticide. Extraordinary because it is not only incredibly effective but it is also very safe. As an insecticide neem can act against over 200 different insect species, as well as many fungal, bacterial, mite and nematode plant infections. Tests in Nigeria have shown that insecticides made from preparations of neem leaves and seeds are as effective as DDT and other highly toxic pesticides. It also kills off the fungus *Aspergillus flavus* which grows on many foods and which is responsible for producing the highly carcinogenic chemicals called aflatoxins.

Neem is as important in treating infections in humans as it is with plants since it is antibacterial, antifungal and antiviral for us too. It has antibacterial activity against *Staphylococcus aureus*, which causes many problems from boils to food poisoning to septicaemia and *Salmonella typhosa*, which causes food poisoning and typhoid. As an antifungal it treats athlete's foot, ringworm and thrush. As an antiviral, neem leaves have long been applied externally to such viral infections as chickenpox, warts and even smallpox. Research shows some evidence for therapeutic effects in hepatitis B and herpes infections.

For many centuries Indians have used neem twigs as makeshift toothbrushes. They pick the twigs, chew the end to soften them – then brush! The antiseptic effects of the tree prevent tooth decay and oral infections and the anti-inflammatory properties of the tree lessen the inflammation of gum disease. When applied to the skin neem stimulates local immune defences and is used to treat eczema, scabies and many other skin problems. Neem extracts also appear to lower blood pressure, lower fevers and have pain-relieving actions. Research is continuing into the traditional claim that this tree can treat malaria.

One of the most fascinating potential uses of neem is the creation of new contraceptive products – for men! Work is currently proceeding to develop an oral contraceptive pill for men to take on the basis that neem oil is an effective spermicide. The oil might also offer a new form of contraception for women as it has strong spermicidal properties when inserted into the vagina before intercourse.

If research helps neem to live up to its promise it will need to be planted on a huge scale. One further gift from the neem is that it has very deep roots that have a special ability to gain nutrition even from poor soils, so they can help to reclaim poor land.

Though not all trees possess the multitude of possibilities that neem presents to us many have substantial gifts to bestow upon us. Looked at in the most holistic sense – both personally and globally, in terms of society and environment, on a human level and a planetary level – tree medicine has much to offer in curing our ills.

PART · TWO

A-Z
of Healing
Trees

Tree Profiles

ABOUT THE PLANT PROFILES

This part of the book contains profiles of individual medicinal trees, outlining their characteristics and uses. Each profile is designed to provide all the essential information needed to help you get to know each tree and understand its healing properties.

The trees are listed alphabetically by their Latin scientific names. This is to avoid confusion. Several different trees are often known by the same common name – at least half a dozen trees are known as Balm of Gilead, and even more are referred to as 'fever tree' – but every tree has its own unique Latin name. You can also look up a tree by its common name by referring to the 'Index of Common Tree Names' (p.303) at the end of the book.

You will notice that some of the profiles are longer than others. This is because there is more information available for some species. These are generally the most medically important and widely used trees. There is also a bias towards the trees that I have most knowledge of using in my own practice. Also, I have given more detailed guidelines on how to use the tree medicines that I have found to be particularly safe and effective according to traditional understanding, research data and my own clinical experience. Each profile gives several types of information – these are listed and described below.

LATIN NAME

Each entry is headed with the plants botanical name. This comes in two parts; the *genus* name comes first followed by the *species* name. For example, with *Crataegus monogyna*, *Crataegus* is the genus name and *monogyna* the species. Several closely related trees may share the same genus name but each individual tree within that genus will have its own unique species name. For instance, *Crataegus monogyna* has a close relative called *Crataegus laevigata*.

COMMON NAME/S

Common names are the names that plants have been given by the communities who have known them. They usually have a descriptive origin, referring to some particular characteristic or attribute of the tree. Any one tree may have many different common names. *Crataegus monogyna* is commonly known by a host of names including bread and cheese, hawthorn, May tree, mother-die, quick-thorn and whitethorn. Such names may vary over very short distances, even between neighbouring villages and a tree may be called by several names within the same locality. These names often have fascinating derivations although their true origins are frequently lost in the mists of time. With *Crataegus monogyna*, 'bread and cheese' is usually taken to describe the taste of the leaves, though some say the leaf is the bread and the fruit is the cheese; 'hawthorn' is now the most frequently used name for this tree and it simply describes its appearance – the fruits (berries) are called haws and the branches bear thorns; 'May tree' reflects the fact that the tree begins flowering in May; 'mother-die' is connected with the belief that bringing *Crataegus monogyna* into the house would presage a death, possibly because the leaves and flowers smell slightly like rotting flesh.

I have just given a few of the most common English names, though occasionally I have provided a non-English name, such as the Zulu name for some African trees and the Spanish or Native names for some South American species.

PLANT FAMILY

Plants are grouped together scientifically by botanists into various families. The members of each family share certain features that link them together. Many families do not contain trees alone but other types of plant as well. Some families are huge, such as the Leguminosae that has at least 16,400 species. Others are very small; an extreme example is the Ginkgoaceae, which has just one surviving member – the gingko tree (*Ginkgo biloba*). To make things more confusing, the names of plant families are sometimes revised by botanists, for example the Leguminosae has also been known as Fabaceae and Papillonaceae.

Related species

I have listed those medicinal tree species closely related to the one being profiled where I think this is useful or interesting. I have not tried to name every related medicinal tree on each occasion.

Not to be confused with

Here, I have sought to clear up some of the common mistakes that occur when identifying medicinal trees. These usually occur where two or more trees share a similar Latin or common name.

Range

This section briefly lists the region where each tree originated and occasionally also gives the places that the tree has spread to, or become 'naturalized' in.

Part/s used

Here I specify which particular part or parts of the tree are used as medicines, such as roots, stem (or trunk), bark, heartwood, twigs, leaves, seeds and fruit. Sometimes a particular extract is used rather than the whole plant part itself. In these cases I have specified the part of the tree from which the extract derives.

Overview

The overview gives a concise summary of each tree. This generally includes a short description of the tree, and details of its history, folklore and non-medical uses, as well as stating its most important therapeutic uses. This section often gives useful treatment tips. You can use this section as a quick reference but, if you do, have a look at the 'Cautions' section as well because this often contains important information not contained in the overview.

Phytochemicals

Phytochemicals are the plants' physiologically active constituents – the ingredients that make tree medicines work. I have avoided giving long lists of chemicals and have just mentioned the main groups, occasionally highlighting an important member of a group. You can find out more about what these chemicals are, and what they do, in Chapter 3.

ACTIONS

The actions section describes what the tree actually does to the body. Some of the terms are readily understandable such as 'immunostimulant' or 'antibacterial'. Others are more difficult. For explanations of these words consult the Glossary at the end of the book.

INDICATIONS

This section details the conditions that the tree is used for. I have mainly listed these using non-technical terms. Some entries for the more widely used herbs have additional notes clarifying how they achieve their benefits. The indications are divided into those conditions to be treated internally and those where the remedy is applied externally. Basically, 'internally' means that the tree medicine is taken by mouth and swallowed; 'externally' means the medicine is given by any other route. By this definition even a gargle or an enema is viewed as being external.

PREPARATION

The preparations are also divided into internal and external use. In most cases no detailed information about how to make the preparations is given since this has already been covered earlier in the book. For description of herbal preparations and for preparations of volatile oils refer to Chapter 4. This book is not intended as a complete home treatment guide and so I have only given specific dosages in a few cases, where the tree medicine is widely used and there is a definite view on how much should be taken. For many trees the dosage range is broad and depends on the condition and the individual who has it – their weight, height, age, constitution, and so on. In general terms, though, other than those trees described as potentially toxic, the dosage terms described along with the preparations on the pages mentioned above can be followed.

CAUTIONS

This is a very important section. As we have said earlier in the book not all tree medicines can be regarded as completely safe. I have pointed out particular cautions where these are known but the absence of a caution against a particular profile does not necessarily mean that the tree can be considered entirely safe.

IMPORTANT

While most of the tree medicines mentioned are safe and gentle, a good number have the potential to cause harm when used in the wrong way or at the wrong dosage. It is advisable to seek expert professional advice before using most tree medicines. You should always inform your doctor if you are taking any alternative forms of medicine. Particular caution should be exercised with vulnerable groups – children, the elderly, in pregnancy and when lactating – if you have a serious medical condition or if you are taking drugs prescribed by a doctor. With regard to volatile oils, these should only be taken internally if on expert professional advice. Avoid undiluted volatile oils coming into direct contact with the skin. Wash your hands immediately after handling volatile oils. As with any medicine, if you are taking any type of tree medicine and you begin to feel unwell, seek expert professional advice.

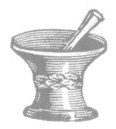

Abies alba

COMMON NAME Silver fir.
PLANT FAMILY Pinaceae.

RELATED SPECIES There are around 40 *Abies* species, several others are used medicinally including *A. balsamea* (balsam fir); *A. grandis* (grand fir). *Pinus* and *Tsuga* trees are members of the same family.

RANGE Europe, Central America.

PARTS USED Bark, needles. The volatile oil extracted from the needles.

OVERVIEW
Firs are a type of pine tree. The silver fir is the tallest European tree and is often grown as a Christmas tree. The volatile oil produced by fir trees is highly antiseptic and is useful as an inhalation or chest rub for thick phlegmy coughs and chest infections. It is also very stimulating to the circulation and helps relieve muscular spasm and pain in rheumatism. It makes a good massage rub for stiff muscles. *A. balsamea* (balsam fir) was used by Native American tribes for the same sorts of problems as those listed below for the silver fir. Several tribes placed the needles in their pillows to ward off infections. Firs are the source of oil of turpentine, which can be distilled down to yield rosin (the resinous substance used by violinists to wax their bows) and also to make varnish and pitch.

Treatment tip – Revitalizing Bath

The volatile oil from fir trees has an excellent stimulating effect on the circulation and is wonderful when added to a hot bath at the end of an exhausting day to revitalize the whole body. Add 5 drops of fir oil to 5ml of sweet almond or olive oil and mix into the bath. Soak for as long as you wish. When you come out of the bath wrap yourself up warmly in bed and rest for half an hour. This is to let the body respond to the rejuvenation that the oil causes. Avoid taking such a bath before bed or you could be kept awake all night!

PHYTOCHEMICALS
Resin, volatile oil.

ACTIONS
Antiseptic, anticatarrhal, circulatory stimulant, expectorant.

INDICATIONS
Externally Respiratory tract infections: chest infections, colds, coughs, sinusitis. Chronic nasal catarrh. Arthritis and rheumatism. Skin boils and infections.

PREPARATIONS

Externally Inhalation of the volatile oil or the steam from an infusion of the needles. A chest rub can be made by diluting the volatile oil in a carrier oil. In arthritis and rheumatism the affected limbs are held over the steam from the infused needles or a poultice of needles was traditionally placed over the area. A fir massage oil can be used instead. The volatile oil added to a cream base can be used for boils and skin infections (such as impetigo).

CAUTIONS

The volatile oil from *Abies* trees has been taken internally (mixed in a capsule with a buffer such as olive oil) to treat severe chest infections such as pneumonia but this should only be done by expert professionals.

Acacia arabica

COMMON NAMES Babul; Indian gum.
PLANT FAMILY Leguminosae.

RELATED SPECIES The Acacia genus is huge! There are around 1,200 species, many of which are used medicinally, including, *A. catechu* (catechu); *A. karroo* (sweet thorn); *A. senegal* (gum arabic); *A. xanthophloea* (fever tree).

RANGE Originates from North Africa, also grown in India and Egypt.

PARTS USED Bark, gum (exuded from the bark), leaves, seeds.

OVERVIEW

Babul has been used as a timber source for buildings as well as being used as a medicine. It grows to around 20m (70ft). Known as 'Indian gum' it is also referred to as gum arabic (though *A. senegal* is the true gum arabic) and gum acacia. It has been used to treat infections of the mouth and to reduce tooth decay. A study designed to investigate the traditional reputation for dental care found that chewing Indian gum helped to reduce plaque levels on teeth. In Ayurvedic medicine, the gum is fried in ghee (clarified butter) and eaten as an aphrodisiac! Gum arabic from *A. senegal* is used in similar ways to Indian gum – externally to soothe wounds, burns and sore nipples, and internally for inflammatory disorders of the stomach, intestines and urinary system as well as coughs.

PHYTOCHEMICALS

Condensed tannins, flavonoids, catechins, mucilage.

ACTIONS

Bark Astringent.
Gum Demulcent.

INDICATIONS
Internally Premature ejaculation (in Ayurvedic medicine), diarrhoea and dysentery.
Externally *Bark* Bleeding gums and gingivitis, conjunctivitis, sore throats.
Gum Coughs, to prevent tooth decay.

PREPARATIONS
Internally Decoction taken by mouth.
Externally Decoction used as a gargle for sore throats, as a mouthwash for bleeding gums, and as an eyebath for conjunctivitis. The gum is chewed to prevent tooth decay or sucked to soothe coughs.

CAUTION
Do not take internally for more than 2–3 weeks at a time.

Acacia catechu

COMMON NAMES Black catechu; cutch.
PLANT FAMILY Leguminosae.

RELATED SPECIES see *Acacia arabica*.

NOT TO BE CONFUSED WITH *Uncaria gambier* (a liana) is also known as catechu (or pale catechu), and *Areca catechu* (betel nut).

RANGE India, Myanmar, Sri Lanka, East Africa.

PARTS USED Bark, heartwood, leaves.

OVERVIEW
Black catechu is a deciduous tree growing to a height of around 25m (80ft), with yellow flowers and typical highly-divided *Acacia* leaves. The heartwood is used for dyeing cloth; it is the original dye used in making khaki cloth. Catechin, one of the main constituents of black catechu, has been shown to be useful in treating hepatitis, it seems to speed up the recovery time for the liver. This tree also helps to lower blood pressure. Traditionally, it has mainly been given as an astringent to bind and heal in disorders where there is discharge of bodily fluids such as diarrhoea, heavy menstrual bleeding and wounds.

PHYTOCHEMICALS
Flavonoids, resins, tannins (including catechin).

ACTIONS
Astringent, coagulant, hypotensive, vulnerary.

INDICATIONS
Internally High blood pressure, heavy menstrual bleeding, diarrhoea, dysentery, hepatitis.
Externally Bleeding gums, ulcers on the skin, sore throat, vaginal discharge, wounds and bleeding.

PREPARATIONS
Internally Decoction. Tincture.
Externally Decoction, used as a douche for vaginal discharge, a wash for wounds, as a mouthwash for bleeding gums and mouth ulcers, and a gargle for sore throats.

CAUTION
Do not take by mouth for more than 2–3 weeks at a time. Pure catechin should not be taken unless under medical supervision as it can cause autoimmune haemolysis (breakdown of red blood cells).

Acer species

COMMON NAME Maple trees.
PLANT FAMILY Aceraceae.

SPECIES USED Many species of maple tree have been used medicinally including *Acer alba* (white maple); *Acer circinatum* (vine maple); *Acer glabrum* (rocky mountain maple); *Acer macrophyllum* (bigleaf maple); *Acer negundo* (box elder); *Acer nigrum* (black maple); *Acer pensylvanicum* (striped maple); *Acer rubrum* (red maple); *Acer saccharinum* (silver maple); *Acer saccharum* (sugar maple); *Acer spicatum* (mountain maple).

RANGE North America.

PARTS USED Bark, leaves, sap, wood (depending on the species).

OVERVIEW
There are more than a hundred *Acer* species and many cultivars grown as ornamental trees for parks and gardens. *Acers* are elegant and graceful with maple-like leaves that display a spectacular range of autumnal colours. Native American tribes have found many uses for these beautiful trees. As well as providing medicines they have also given foods (most famously the delicious maple syrup from the sugar maple), dyes, fuel and wood for making arrows and children's toys. As traditional medicines in

North America they treated a wide range of health problems from coughs to pains. Recently, an extract from sugar maple sap has found favour as an ingredient in skin care products. It soothes, nourishes and moisturises the skin.

PHYTOCHEMICALS
Tannins, polysaccharides.

ACTIONS
This depends on the species and the following is just a selection: Antihaemorrhagic (*Acer spicatum*), astringent (*Acer circinatum*), expectorant (*Acer alba*), galactagogue (*Acer glabrum*), spasmolytic (*Acer saccharinum*).

INDICATIONS
This depends on the species and includes:
Internally Colds (*Acer pensylvanicum* bark), coughs (*Acer saccharinum* bark, *Acer saccharum* bark, *Acer alba* bark), cramping pains (*Acer rubrum* bark, *Acer saccharinum* bark), diarrhoea (*Acer nigrum* inner bark, *Acer circinatum* wood), to stimulate milk flow in breastfeeding mothers (*Acer glabrum* twigs).
Externally Abscesses (*Acer spicatum* root chips).

PREPARATIONS
Internally Bark, twigs and root chips are prepared by decoction.
Externally Poultices.

CAUTIONS
None found.

Acokanthera oppositifolia

COMMON NAME Poison-bush; uhlunguyembe (Zulu).
PLANT FAMILY Apocynaceae.

RELATED SPECIES *A. oblongifolia; A. schimperi.*

RANGE Africa.

PARTS USED leaves, roots, wood.

OVERVIEW
Poison-bush is a small evergreen tree growing up to 5m (15ft) tall, though it often occurs as a shrub. Its common name derives from the fact that this tree contains ouabain which has been used as an arrow poison for hunting; it can cause death within 20 minutes of entering the bloodstream. It is used by Maasai

hunters in Kenya. In conventional medicine ouabain can be given as an injection to help treat some cases of heart failure. Traditionally, this plant has been given to induce vomiting to rid the body of the poison from snakebites and is used generally to relieve pain.

PHYTOCHEMICALS
Cardiac glycosides including ouabain. (*A. schimperi* is also used as an arrow poison, acolongifloroside K being the major active constituent in the poison alongside ouabain).

ACTIONS
Analgesic, cardioactive, emetic.

INDICATIONS
Internally The tree has traditionally been used to treat headaches, snakebites (leaves and root); stomach pain, toothache (leaves).

PREPARATIONS
Internally Traditionally, weak infusions of the leaves have been used most commonly in order to keep the toxic components to low levels.

CAUTIONS
The poison-bush is potentially precisely that! Although it may be of value in skilled hands when given at the correct dosage its general use should be avoided.

Adansonia digitata

COMMON NAMES Baobab, Judas's bag, monkey bread (English);
muvhuyu, shimuwu (African).
PLANT FAMILY Bombacaceae.

RELATED SPECIES *Adansonia gregorii* (gourd tree).

RANGE Africa.

PARTS USED Bark, dried fruit pulp, (occasionally leaves and seeds).

Amazing trees

The wonderfully named baobab is an extraordinary tree. It can live for over 2,000 years and the trunk can develop a massive circumference (this can be more than 20m/65ft).

OVERVIEW

The bark of the baobab lies smooth over the muscular growth of the wood, and the tree is very short in relation to its girth. This gives fully-matured trees the appearance of a kind of squat, many-armed monster! The baobab has many uses. The bark is made into cloth and rope, the fruit and seeds are used for fuel, the fruit feeds animals and the wood is used for construction. The powdery pulp gathered around the seeds is known as cream of tartare; the Afrikaan name for the tree is kremetart. It is used in African medicine for fevers and diarrhoea. It is also grown in India and used in Ayurvedic medicine internally for fevers (including night sweats associated with tuberculosis) and externally for skin diseases and rheumatism.

PHYTOCHEMICALS

Betulinic acid, flavonols, citric acid (fruit pulp).

ACTIONS

Antifungal , anti-inflammatory, diaphoretic.

INDICATIONS

Internally Diarrhoea, fever, urinary problems.

PREPARATIONS

Internally Bark and leaves by decoction; the fruit pulp is taken mixed with water.

CAUTIONS

None found.

Adhatoda vasica

(also known as *Justicia adhatoda*)
COMMON NAME Malabar nut tree.
PLANT FAMILY Acanthaceae.

RANGE India, Sri Lanka.

PARTS USED Leaves principally (also root, flowers, fruit).

OVERVIEW

The Malabar nut tree is an evergreen that grows mainly in the lower Himalayas. It acts principally on the respiratory system and the drug bromhexine (Bisolvon) was developed from its main alkaloid. It is used to treat asthma because it acts on the three main problems caused by this disorder – it opens up narrowed airways in the lungs (bronchodilator), helps to bring up phlegm (expectorant), and counters the allergic reaction involved in this condition.

PHYTOCHEMICALS
Alkaloids (principally vasicine), volatile oil.

ACTIONS
Antiallergic, bronchodilator, expectorant, oxytocic.

INDICATIONS
Internally Asthma, bronchitis, post-partum haemorrhage (bleeding following childbirth).
Externally Gum disease.

PREPARATIONS
Internally Decoction or tincture of the leaves. They are also smoked to relieve asthma.
Externally Decoction of the leaves as a mouthwash for gum disorders.

CAUTION
None found.

Aegle marmelos

COMMON NAMES Bengal quince; bael; golden apple.
PLANT FAMILY Rutaceae.

RANGE India, Myanmar.

PARTS USED Fruit, bark.

OVERVIEW
This tree is sacred to Hindus. The wood is used as timber, the flowers for scenting water, the unripe fruit provides a yellow dye and the bark produces a gum. Medicinally it has traditionally been used mainly for bowel disorders and as a nutritious convalescent food.

PHYTOCHEMICALS
Fruit Ascorbic acid, beta-carotene, calcium, iron, fibre, niacin, thiamine, potassium, protein, riboflavin, mucilage, pectin, tannin.
Bark Fagarine, marmin, tannin.

ACTIONS
Astringent, hypoglycaemic, nutritive.

> ### New research
>
> Aegle marmelos has recently been shown to be of possible use in controlling diabetes. Also, a clinical trial of an Ayurvedic medicine containing Aegle marmelos and Bacopa monniere showed improvements in symptoms of irritable bowel syndrome (especially when diarrhoea was a prominent feature).

INDICATIONS

Internally The half-ripe fruit is used to treat dysentery and diarrhoea while the ripe fruit is given for constipation. The fruit may be of value in treating non-insulin-dependent diabetes and irritable bowel syndrome. It is taken as a restorative in convalescence, to aid recovery from illness.

PREPARATIONS

Internally The fresh fruit is used either as a decoction or by eating the fruit pulp.

CAUTIONS

None found.

Aesculus hippocastanum

COMMON NAMES Horse chestnut; white chestnut.
PLANT FAMILY Hippocastanaceae.

RELATED SPECIES *A. californica* (California buckeye); *A. x carnea* (red horse chestnut); *A. pavia* (red buckeye).

NOT TO BE CONFUSED WITH *Castanea sativa* (sweet chestnut). Sweet chestnuts are edible, horse chestnuts are not.

RANGE Eurasia.

PARTS USED The seed (conker) principally, though the bark was formerly used.

OVERVIEW

The horse chestnut is a stately tree with large divided leaves and spectacular spikes of white flowers (tinged with yellow or pink at the base of the petals) known as candles. The seeds are used in medicine and they come packaged in round prickly shells. The seeds themselves are called conkers and are still used to play the game that involves bashing one conker against another to see which can avoid disintegration for the longest time (a World Conker Championship is held annually in England!). The horse chestnut, as its name suggests, was used to treat horses for chest conditions, principally coughs. In humans, preparations of the seed have proven effective in treating problems caused by impaired blood supply in the veins. They alleviate symptoms of heaviness, tingling, pain, itching, tiredness and coldness associated with poor circulation in the legs. The combined effect is one of strengthening the small blood vessel walls by decreasing the size and quantity of their pores. This means that horse chestnut is very helpful for treating varicose veins, swollen legs (due to venous problems) and piles. More recently, external use as a cream or ointment has shown beneficial effects on the skin, strengthening the skin cells and helping with medical and cosmetic problems such as cellulite and ageing of the skin. The bark was used to treat fevers and externally applied for ulcers but it has fallen out of use in recent years. Native American tribes have used several *Aesculus* species for a variety of conditions. *A. californica* was used by the Costanoan and Kawaiisu tribes for haemorrhoids and the Mendocino used the bark for toothaches.

Flower remedy

Horse chestnut provides two of the Bach flower remedies: 'chestnut bud' is given to treat the psychological state of 'those who do not take full advantage of observation and experience, and who take a longer time than others to learn the lessons of daily life'; 'white chestnut', made from the flowers, is taken by 'those who cannot prevent thoughts, ideas, arguments which they do not desire entering their minds'. One of the horse chestnut's hybrids, *Aesculus x carnea* (red horse chestnut), provides another of the flower remedies, red chestnut, for 'those who find it difficult not to be anxious for other people'. This tree is not used in traditional medicine but is widely planted as an ornamental in parks and gardens.

PHYTOCHEMICALS
Flavonoids, saponins (aescin), sterols.

ACTIONS
Anti-inflammatory, venous trophorestorative.

INDICATIONS
Internally and externally Bruises, haemorrhoids (piles), varicose veins, swelling (oedema) of the ankles and legs due to problems with veins.
Externally To treat poor skin tone, cellulite and the effects of ageing.

PREPARATIONS

Internally The tincture is the best preparation to take by mouth. Tablets are also available. Two Bach Flower Remedies (chestnut bud and white chestnut) can be taken for the psychological state.

Externally Horse chestnut cream or ointment.

CAUTIONS

Externally it should not be used on broken skin as the saponins may cause irritation. Otherwise horse chestnut is considered to be safe and well tolerated.

Ailanthus altissima

COMMON NAME Tree of heaven; tree of the gods; Chinese sumach.
PLANT FAMILY Simaroubaceae.

RELATED SPECIES *A. malabarica*; *A. vilmoriniana*. *Picrasma excelsa* (quassia) and *Quassia amara* (Surinam quassia wood) are members of the same family.

RANGE Originating in China, naturalized to North America and Central and Southern Europe.

PARTS USED Inner part of the bark, the extracted resin, roots.

OVERVIEW

This large (25m/80ft) attractive deciduous Chinese tree was cultivated in Europe as an ornamental species from the eigthteenth century. It grows rapidly and has ash-like leaves which grow 1–2 feet (30–60cm) long. Its wood is used for cabinet making and it has been planted along streets in towns. The towering beauty of this tree, when fully mature, is reflected in its common name – tree of heaven. It has traditionally been used for heart and chest problems as well as for dysentery and diarrhoea. Research has revealed that it contains compounds that may be of use in treating tuberculosis.

PHYTOCHEMICALS

Lignin, resin, tannins.

ACTIONS

Antispasmodic, astringent.

INDICATIONS

Internally Dysentery, asthma, heart palpitations.

PREPARATIONS
Internally Decoction of the stem bark for dysentery; tincture of the root bark for asthma and palpitations.

CAUTIONS
None found.

Albizia lebbeck

COMMON NAME East Indian walnut; kokko; siris.
PLANT FAMILY Leguminosae.

RELATED SPECIES Several *Albizia* species are used medicinally, including *A. anthelmintica*; *A. adianthifolia* (flat-crown); *A. julibrissin* (silk tree); *A. odoratissima*.

RANGE Originating in Asia but naturalized in the Caribbean and Africa.

PART USED Stem bark.

OVERVIEW
Research has shown that the East Indian walnut tree has antiallergic properties. It stabilizes the body's mast cells (which are one of the mediators of inflammation) and allergy-causing antibodies. This activity makes it useful in the related group of atopic (allergic) disorders – asthma, hayfever and eczema. Both East Indian walnut and a related species, *A. anthelmintica*, have been shown to lower cholesterol levels. The latter species is used by African tribes who add it to the pot when cooking meat. It appears to prevent the negative effects of meat fats on their health. This species is also given to treat worm infestation. *A. adianthifolia* is utilized for skin disorders and headaches. *A. julibrissin* is taken for insomnia, boils and poor memory. *A. odoratissima* is used in India for leprosy and ulcers.

PHYTOCHEMICALS
Saponins, cardiac glycosides, tannins, flavonoids.

ACTIONS
Antifungal, antibacterial, hypocholesterolaemic, antiallergic.

INDICATIONS
Internally Asthma, eczema, allergic rhinitis (hayfever), to prevent and treat high cholesterol levels.
Externally Eczema.

PREPARATIONS
Internally Decoction of the bark or tincture taken by mouth.

Externally Decoction or tincture applied directly onto affected areas of the skin in eczema.

CAUTIONS
None found.

Alnus glutinosa

COMMON NAME Black alder; common alder; European alder.
PLANT FAMILY Betulaceae.

NOT TO BE CONFUSED WITH Alder buckthorn (*Frangula alnus*).

RANGE Eurasia, the Mediterranean.

PARTS USED Bark, leaves.

OVERVIEW
The common alder is a handsome deciduous tree. Several ornamental cultivars are available. The wood has been important in the manufacture of clogs, boats, buildings, gunpowder charcoal and (it is said) Stradivarius violins. Alder was used to provide the underpinnings (piles) for Venice since it does not rot in water. The tree itself likes to grow in wet places. It is popular for carving and in cultivation it can be coppiced, providing poles for fencing and other purposes. The bark is used to tan hides, giving leather a red colour. It is used medically as an astringent but was also traditionally employed in treating malaria and rheumatism. A reference from Norfolk, England refers to the leaves being lightly bruised and applied to heal burns.

PHYTOCHEMICALS
Bark Tannins, lignans, phenolic glycosides.
Leaves Flavonoid glycosides, resin.

ACTIONS
Astringent, possible anti-inflammatory.

INDICATIONS
Externally Sore throats, mouth ulcers, bruises and swellings.

PREPARATIONS
Externally Decoction as a gargle for sore throats, a mouthwash for mouth ulcers, and applied as a compress to bruises and swellings.

CAUTIONS
None found.

Alstonia scholaris

COMMON NAME Dita bark; devil tree; milky pine.
PLANT FAMILY Apocynaceae.

RELATED SPECIES *A. macrophylla*; *A. constricta* (fever bark).

RANGE South-east Asian rainforests.

PART USED Bark.

OVERVIEW
The wood of this evergreen tree was used for making writing slates, which leads to its species name – *scholaris*. It has been utilized traditionally to deter insects and has a reputed action in treating malaria and rheumatism. A large tree, it grows 12–18m (40–60ft) in height. The bark of an Australian species (*A. constricta*) was also used to treat malaria and has been called 'Australian quinine'. It remains one of the most important fever trees and bitter tonics in Australian medicine and is also used to treat high blood pressure.

New research

Research into this tree has shown that it protects the liver from damage by toxins. Studies have also shown that extracts from another *Alstonia* species, *A. macrophylla*, have antitumour effects against experimental cancer cell lines and activity against *Plasmodium falciparum*, one of the causes of malaria.

PHYTOCHEMICALS
Betulinic acid; indole alkaloids (including akuammidine, echitamine).

ACTIONS
Febrifuge, hypotensive, spasmolytic.

INDICATIONS
Internally Diarrhoea and dysentery; possibly malaria and high blood pressure.

PREPARATIONS
Internally Decoctions of the bark.

CAUTIONS
Alstonia species should be taken on expert professional advice only. They can stimulate the uterus and should be avoided in pregnancy.

Anacardium occidentale

COMMON NAMES Cashew nut tree; Acajou; Cajueiro.
PLANT FAMILY Anacardiaceae.

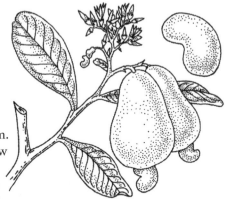

RANGE Originating from tropical America, grown in Africa.

PARTS USED Bark, gum (from the trunk), leaves, nuts.

OVERVIEW
Cashew nuts are a popular food item. They are borne within the small cashew fruit, which has a curious appearance because it has the bean-like shape of the nut and is suspended below the fruit peduncle, which is larger than the fruit itself. This swollen peduncle (the bit that attaches the fruit to the tree) is known as the 'cashew apple' and is edible. Its juice is rich in vitamin C and is used to treat influenza. Several other parts of the tree are used in medicine. A gum obtained from the trunk treats bacterial, fungal and parasite infections. A study showed that cashew extract was effective against a wide range of bacteria including *E. coli*. The leaves are used for malaria and toothache. The bark is taken by some rainforest tribes as a contraceptive. The bark has been given as a treatment for diabetes.

PHYTOCHEMICALS
Alkaloids (leaves); anacardic acid (in the gum); fats and protein (nuts); tannins (bark and leaves); vitamins and minerals ('fruit' and nuts).

ACTIONS
Antimicrobial (gum); possible antiviral or immunostimulant (peduncle juice); possible contraceptive (bark); nutritive (nuts).

INDICATIONS
Internally Asthma (bark); diarrhoea (bark and leaves); malaria, toothache (leaves); worm infestation (gum); nourishing restorative in convalescence (nuts).
Externally Fungal skin infections (gum).

PREPARATIONS
Internally The nuts are eaten. Decoction of bark, gum and leaves.
Externally Decoction of gum.

CAUTIONS
The oil lining the shell of the cashew nut is an irritant.

Andira araroba

COMMON NAME Araroba; Goa powder.
PLANT FAMILY Leguminosae.

RELATED SPECIES *A. inermis* (cabbage tree); *A. parviflora*.

RANGE South America, especially Brazil.

PARTS USED Branches, stem.

OVERVIEW
Andira araroba is a large South American tree that gives a yellow powder from its branches and stem, known as Goa powder. Taken by mouth this causes vomiting and diarrhoea. Because of this it has been used as a rather unpleasant traditional 'cleansing' treatment for skin problems such as acne, eczema and psoriasis. It is also used externally as an ointment for the same problems. Its principal use today is for parasitic skin disorders.

PHYTOCHEMICALS
Anthraquinone complex (known as chrysarobin).

ACTIONS
Antiparasitic, cathartic, evacuant.

INDICATIONS
Internally Acne, eczema, psoriasis.
Externally Acne, eczema, psoriasis, ringworm, scabies.

PREPARATIONS
Externally As an ointment for skin disorders.

CAUTIONS
Do not take internally, may cause vomiting and digestive tract disturbance.

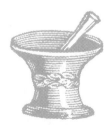

Annona squamosa

COMMON NAME   Custard apple; sweet sop.
PLANT FAMILY   Annonaceae.

RELATED SPECIES   Many *Annona* species are used medicinally including *A. bullata*; *A. cherimola* (cherimoya); *A. muricata* (guanabana, sour sop); *A. reticulata* (bullock's heart, wild custard apple); *A. senegalensis*.

NOT TO BE CONFUSED WITH   *Asimina triloba* is also commonly known as custard apple.

RANGE   Tropical America.

PARTS USED   Fruits, leaves, seeds.

OVERVIEW

The curiously named custard apple tree grows up to 10m (30ft) tall. The fruits are edible. The leaves were used for 'dropsy' (swollen feet connected with heart failure); they contain an alkaloid that stimulates heart activity, helping it to perform better when it is failing. Research into the bark has revealed several compounds (including acetogenins) that have anticancer properties. Other *Annona* species have medical uses such as *A. bullata* and *A. montana* (potential anticancer activity); *A. muricata* (potential use in malaria).

PHYTOCHEMICALS

Alkaloids (including higenamine); mucilage.

ACTIONS

Astringent, diuretic (leaves); carminative (seeds).

INDICATIONS

Internally Colds and fevers, diarrhoea, dysentery.

PREPARATIONS

Internally Decoction.

CAUTIONS

To be used on expert professional advice only. Alkaloids from *Annona* plants have been shown to affect brain structures in animal experiments. It has been suggested that there may be a link between consuming *A. squamosa* and *A. muricata* and an increased incidence of unusual forms of Parkinson's disease.

Aquilaria malaccensis

COMMON NAME Agarwood; eaglewood; aloewood; calambac.
PLANT FAMILY Thymelaeaceae.

RELATED SPECIES *A. sinensis.*

RANGE Indo-Malaysia.

PARTS USED Bark, heartwood, resin.

Conservation

Both *A. malaccensis* and *A. sinensis* are classed as being vulnerable to extinction in the wild in the medium term due to exploitation for medicinal use. *A. malaccensis* is considered critically endangered in India where its export is banned.

OVERVIEW

This tree is the aloe referred to in the Bible, but it is most often referred to as agarwood. Its resin is used as incense and in manufacturing perfumes; it has a smell resembling sandalwood. Medically it is principally used for digestive and lung problems and fevers. Research has revealed that the bark contains anticancer compounds.

PHYTOCHEMICALS

Anticancer chemicals.

ACTIONS

Antispasmodic, astringent, tonic to the digestive system.

INDICATIONS

Internally Asthma, bronchitis, coughs, indigestion, digestive spasms, rheumatism, fevers.

PREPARATIONS

Internally Decoctions of the bark and heartwood.

CAUTIONS

None found.

Areca catechu

COMMON NAMES Betel nut; areca nut.
PLANT FAMILY Arecaceae.

NOT TO BE CONFUSED WITH *Acacia catechu* (black catechu).

RANGE cultivated in India, Bangladesh, Ceylon, West Malaysia, the Philippines, Japan.

PARTS USED Fruit rind, seeds (nuts).

OVERVIEW
This attractive tree has yellowish fruits containing a single seed traditionally used in Ayurvedic and Chinese medicine. Orientals also chew the seeds (betel nuts) as an exhilarating stimulant. This habit has been associated with cancer of the mouth (though the seed is sometimes mixed with tobacco for chewing and this may partially explain the problem). Medicinally it has been used principally to treat worm infestations.

PHYTOCHEMICALS
Alkaloids (including arecoline); tannins; fixed oil.

ACTIONS
Antiparasitic, appetite suppressant, astringent, cardiac stimulant (seeds); diuretic, laxative (fruit rind).

INDICATIONS
Internally Constipation (fruit rind); dysentery, parasite infestation, malaria (seeds).

PREPARATIONS
Internally Decoction of seeds or fruit rind.

CAUTIONS
The nuts should not be chewed because of the link with oral cancer. The seeds can cause vomiting, increased saliva production and intoxication. They can also blacken the teeth.

Aspidosperma species

COMMON NAME Depends on species.
PLANT FAMILY Apocynaceae.

SPECIES USED There are around 80 *Aspidosperma* species, many of which are medicinal, including, *A. nitidum*; *A. excelsum*; *A. marcgravianum*; *A. quebracho-blanco (quebracho)*; *A. tomentosum*; *A. schultesii*.

RANGE South America; West Indies.

PARTS USED Bark, latex, leaves, roots.

OVERVIEW

Aspidosperma are evergreen trees varying in size from small to large depending on the species. As a group they are very rich in alkaloids, which means they generally have strong effects on the body's functioning. Some species are capable of killing infective organisms. *Aspidosperma quebracho-blanco* (meaning 'hard white wood') was used by the American Eclectic medical practitioners in the early twentieth century to treat shortness of breath due to heart disease and asthma, and in malarial fevers. This species is also said to be an aphrodisiac (it contains alkaloids similar to those present in the famed aphrodisiac tree yohimbe).

PHYTOCHEMICALS

Alkaloids; tannins.

ACTIONS

(depending on species)
Antimicrobial, aphrodisiac, febrifuge.

INDICATIONS

Internally Difficulties with respiration; fevers; impotence.
Externally Skin infections.

PREPARATIONS

Internally Decoction of the dried bark or leaves.
Externally The latex applied externally to infected skin areas.

CAUTIONS

Not for general use. Only to be used on expert professional advice to avoid toxicity. Overdose causes vomiting.

Azadirachta indica

COMMON NAME Neem tree.
PLANT FAMILY Meliaceae.

RANGE Native to India, it is common throughout Asia and parts of Africa.

PARTS USED Bark, leaves, seed oil.

OVERVIEW
This is an evergreen tree growing to 30m (100ft) tall. It has an extraordinary range of known and potential uses. Neem has many medical uses but also provides fuel, timber, cosmetics and fertilizers. It is being studied as a major source of pesticides. Medical use includes treating a variety of infections, skin diseases and dental problems. It also has a role to play as a contraceptive. This is a truly remarkable tree, being one of the most versatile and beneficent known.

Treatment tip – Scabies

A study has shown an extract of the bark to have significant anti-fungal activity against *Candida* infection. In a trial on 814 people with scabies using a paste of neem and turmeric (*Curcuma longa*) the treatment was effective in 97% of cases within 3–15 days; the authors concluded this to be a safe and effective treatment.

PHYTOCHEMICALS
Limonoids (these are triterpenes, including azadarachtin).

ACTIONS
Anodyne, antibacterial, antifungal, anti-inflammatory, antipyretic, antiseptic, antiviral.

INDICATIONS
Family planning There is a potential role of using neem as a form of birth control in men and women.
Parasite infestations Neem has been used in Chaga's disease and malaria.
Skin diseases Athlete's foot, boils, eczema, head lice, infected ulcers, psoriasis, ringworm, scabies, warts.
Teeth and gums Neem has a role in prevention of tooth decay and diseases of the teeth and gums.

PREPARATIONS
Internally Decoction of leaves, taken by mouth.

Externally Neem extracts are used in several toothpastes and other dental products. The sticks are chewed and used as makeshift toothbrushes. Leaf poultice applied to skin disorders. Oil is applied to the hair to kill head lice or to cure skin disorders.

CAUTIONS

Neem tree is generally considered safe and non-toxic apart from the seed oil. However, there are reports that prolonged drinking of the leaf tea may cause liver and kidney damage. It is not advised to take the oil by mouth (although toxic effects of the oil may be due to contamination rather than to the oil itself).

Bertholletia excelsa

COMMON NAMES Brazil nut.
PLANT FAMILY Lecythidaceae.

RANGE Amazon Basin.

PARTS USED Nut, seed oil.

OVERVIEW

The Brazil nut tree is one of the tallest of all rainforest trees, growing up to 45m (150ft). It has large fruits, which contain about 20 hard-shelled seeds (Brazil nuts). The economic value of Brazil nuts as a rainforest product is second only to rubber. The extracted oil is used for cooking, as lamp fuel and for manufacturing soap. Brazil nuts have been in the limelight more recently as a prime source of the trace mineral selenium. Just one nut gives more than the recommended daily allowance for this nutrient. If you have low selenium levels you may be at greater risk of cancer, heart disease and premature ageing. Supplementing the diet with Brazil nuts may help reduce the risk of these problems. Selenium also improves fertility in men and seems to reduce the risk of miscarriage. Low levels of selenium are connected with depression and other psychiatric disorders. It truly is a remarkable nutrient and because of its importance in so many areas, including fertility, cancer prevention, psychological health and the immune system, it makes good sense to supplement the diet with Brazil nuts on a daily basis. The bark is traditionally boiled for liver diseases. Unfortunately, Brazil nuts are usually harvested from the wild in a way that is unsustainable. Try and buy Brazil nuts from suppliers who can guarantee that they are collecting the nuts ethically.

PHYTOCHEMICALS

Oils (including oleic, palmitic, linoleic and alpha linolenic acids); protein – amino acids (including cysteine, methionine); selenium.

ACTIONS

Antioxidant, immunostimulant, nutritive.

INDICATIONS

Internally As a general nutritional supplement possibly having a role in preventing some types of cancer and stimulating immune function therefore protecting against infection. Depression and infertility.

PREPARATIONS

Internally The nuts are eaten as they are, or used in cooking. One nut a day provides an excellent selenium supplement. The bark is decocted.

CAUTIONS

The nuts are a common and well tolerated food item. No adverse effects of the bark have been found.

Betula pendula

COMMON NAMES Birch; silver birch.
PLANT FAMILY Betulaceae.

RELATED SPECIES *B. alleghaniensis* (yellow birch); *B. lenta* (American black birch), the distilled oil is rich in methyl salicylate; *B. papyrifera* (paper birch); *B. pubescens* (downy birch); *B. utilis*.

RANGE Europe.

PARTS USED Bark; leaf buds; leaves; sap (tapped from the trunk).

OVERVIEW

The silver birch is an elegant, graceful tree. It has fine delicate branches and leaves that move easily in the wind. The smooth and papery silver bark is distinctive and large stands of birches in autumn are a glorious vision. Birch tar oil is made from the bark. The sap is taken from the trunk of the tree and is popular for making birch wine. The main parts of the plant used medicinally however are the leaves, either gathered in bud or when fully opened. They are diuretic and anti-inflammatory, providing benefits in joint diseases such as arthritis and gout. They are rich in potassium so they do not cause the potassium-depleting problem associated with conventional diuretic drugs. In gout they are particularly useful as they help to decrease the levels of uric acid in the body, which causes this condition.

PHYTOCHEMICALS

Flavonoids (including hyperoside, quercetin); resins; saponins; tannins; volatile oil.

Treatment tip – Gout

If you suffer from gout you can drink birch leaf tea on a regular basis as a preventive medicine. It also helps to follow a diet that excludes purine-containing foods since these contribute to raising uric acid levels. Avoid eating red meat, especially organ meats, seafood, lentils and beans.

ACTIONS
Anti-inflammatory, diuretic, laxative, decreases uric acid levels.

INDICATIONS
Internally Arhtritis, eczema, gout, kidney and bladder disorders (such as cystitis, kidney stones); rheumatism (muscular pain), psoriasis.
Externally Eczema, psoriasis.

PREPARATIONS
Internally
Juice A juice pressed from the fresh leaves is available, taken at 10ml twice a day, in water.
Sap Taken fresh or preserved with alcohol as a diuretic and anti-inflammatory.
Tea Infusion of the leaves is taken 3 to 4 times a day. The tea is pleasantly aromatic and refreshing.
Tincture
Externally
Ointment An ointment is made with birch tar oil and applied externally to psoriasis and eczema patches as required.

CAUTIONS
None found.

Bixa orellana

COMMON NAME Annatto.
PLANT FAMILY Bixaceae.

RANGE Tropical America.

PARTS USED Leaves, fruits, roots, seeds, shoots.

OVERVIEW
Although frequently found as a bush, annatto can grow as a small tree up to 5m (15ft) tall. The seed capsules are strikingly colourful being either a strong red or vivid yellow. The seeds themselves give an orange/red dye used for clothing and

other fabrics and as body paint by native peoples. The dye is still employed widely for cosmetics and in food colouring. Several parts of annatto have been used to treat a wide range of health problems such as sexually transmitted diseases, hepatitis, and skin disorders. Annatto seeds may be of benefit in controlling cholesterol levels and high blood pressure.

PHYTOCHEMICALS
Carotenoid pigments (bixin), flavonoids, saponins, tannins.

ACTIONS
Antibacterial (leaves, fruits, shoots); antioxidant, expectorant (seeds); astringent (leaves); febrifuge (shoots); hepatoprotective.

INDICATIONS
Internally Diarrhoea, dysentery (leaves and shoots); hepatitis, prostatitis, skin disorders (leaves); fevers, sexually transmitted disease (shoots); coughs and chest disorders, high cholesterol (seeds); hypertension (roots and seeds).

PREPARATIONS
Internally
Leaves, roots, shoots Decoction.
Seed Decoction or dried and taken as a powder.

CAUTIONS
None found.

Boswellia species

COMMON NAME Frankincense; olibanum; salai guggal.
PLANT FAMILY Burseraceae.

SPECIES USED *B. sacra* (frankincense); *B. frereana* (African elemi); *B. serrata* (salai guggal).

RANGE North-east Africa, Somalia, India.

PART USED Gum-resin.

OVERVIEW
The resins of *Boswellia* trees have been used widely as medicines and for incense. The most famous of these is the frankincense of the Bible. The main medicinal species is *Boswellia serrata*. It is recognized for its value in treating asthma and arthritis.

PHYTOCHEMICALS
Gum-resin (containing boswellic acids).

ACTIONS
Anti-inflammatory, circulatory stimulant.

INDICATIONS
Internally Asthma, inflammatory disorders
(including osteo- and rheumatoid arthritis,
inflammatory bowel disease).

PREPARATIONS
Internally Tincture or a standardized extract
based on boswellic acids at 200–400mg three
times a day.

CAUTIONS
Resinous preparations can cause digestive irritation
or pain. This tendency can be lessened by always taking
them diluted with water and with meals.

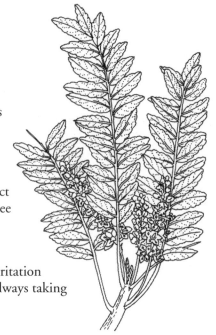

Brunfelsia grandiflora

COMMON NAME Fever tree; chiric sanango.
PLANT FAMILY Solanaceae.

RELATED SPECIES *B. chiricaspi*; *B. uniflorus*.

NOT TO BE CONFUSED WITH Many trees are known as 'fever tree'.

RANGE Tropical South America.

PARTS USED Bark, leaves, roots.

OVERVIEW
Brunfelsia grandiflora is a small rainforest tree with pretty purple flowers. As its
common name suggests this is one of several trees with a reputation for treating
fevers (including yellow fever). Additionally, it has been given for syphilis,
snakebite poisonings, and joint disorders (arthritis and rheumatism). It is also
taken as an hallucinogen, either on its own or as part of preparations containing
ayahuasca (*Banisteriopsis caapi*, a liana). It is used by South American tribes as
part of ceremonies and rituals and by shamans as an aid to diagnosis (contacting
the spirit world).

PHYTOCHEMICALS
Alkaloids, furocoumarin (scopoletin).

ACTIONS

Abortifacient, anti-inflammatory, diuretic, diaphoretic, hallucinogenic.

INDICATIONS

Internally Arthritis, fevers, sexually transmitted disease.

PREPARATIONS

Internally The root is the part used most frequently, prepared by decoction.

CAUTIONS

Due to its hallucinogenic effects this tree should not be used as a medicine unless upon expert professional advice. It should not be used in pregnancy as it is reported to cause abortions.

Buxus sempervirens

COMMON NAME Box; European box.
PLANT FAMILY Buxaceae.

NOT TO BE CONFUSED WITH *Cornus florida* is sometimes known as American boxwood.

RANGE Europe and the Mediterranean.

PARTS USED Leaves, wood.

OVERVIEW

Although capable of growing as a small tree, box is most often encountered as a cultivated hedge. It is often found providing low neatly-clipped borders in ornamental herb gardens or as the main framework for knot gardens. It is an evergreen and has very hard wood that has been put to such uses as making musical instruments and in carving. Its dark and sombre appearance, together with its evergreen habit and longevity, have led to it being planted in graveyards and used in burial rituals. Although once used quite widely in medicine, box is now seldom utilized due to its high level of toxicity. The major interest recently has lain in the potential that a box extract may have a role in delaying the progression of HIV to AIDS.

PHYTOCHEMICALS

Alkaloids (known as buxine).

ACTIONS

Cathartic, diaphoretic, emetic, sedative.

INDICATIONS
Internally It was formerly used for malaria, rheumatism and syphilis.
Externally To improve hair growth.

PREPARATIONS
Internally The leaves or wood were formerly taken as decoctions by mouth. A special extract, SPV30, has been used internally in trials for HIV/AIDS.
Externally Decoction applied as a wash to improve hair growth.

CAUTIONS
Box is highly toxic and should only be used under expert professional advice. It can cause abdominal pain and vomiting and may prove fatal.

Calycophyllum spruceanum

COMMON NAME Firewood tree; capirona; mulateiro; palo mulato.
PLANT FAMILY Rubiaceae.

RELATED SPECIES *C. acreanum*; *C. obovatum*.

RANGE Tropical America.

PART USED Bark.

OVERVIEW
This is a large tree (up to 30m/100ft) with peeling, papery bark. It is used for fuel and to make charcoal. Medically it is applied to skin infections and taken for diabetes. It is sometimes found as one the ingredients in hallucinogenic ayahuasca formulae.

PHYTOCHEMICALS
Possibly alkaloids; tannins.

ACTIONS
Anthelmintic, antifungal, antiseptic, possible hypoglycaemic.

INDICATIONS
Internally Diabetes.
Externally Fungal and parasite skin infections; wounds.

PREPARATIONS
Internally Decoction taken by mouth for diabetes.
Externally Decocted or powdered bark applied to the skin.

CAUTIONS
None found.

Cananga odorata

COMMON NAME Ylang ylang.
PLANT FAMILY Annonaceae.

RANGE Indonesia, the Philippines.

PARTS USED Volatile oil distilled from the flowers (or sometimes the leaves).

OVERVIEW
Ylang ylang means 'flower of flowers' and this tree is famed for its scent, which is used in the perfume industry as well as in medicine. The volatile oil is used widely by aromatherapists as a calming and sensual agent. It is viewed as an aphrodisiac. It may help with impotence and reduced sexual interest when applied as a massage oil or evaporated as a room fragrance. Be a little cautious though, ylang ylang is not to everyone's taste and some find the scent too soapy or cloying. The flowers have been taken internally for malaria.

PHYTOCHEMICALS
Volatile oil Hydrocarbons; alcohols (especially linalool); esters; ethers.

ACTIONS
Antipyretic, antiseptic, anxiolytic, hypotensive, sedative.

INDICATIONS
Externally Anxiety, stress, and generally where relaxation is required. As a massage oil it may be of value in cases of lowered libido and impotence of psychological origin. High blood pressure.

PREPARATIONS
Externally The volatile oil used as a room fragrance and as a massage oil (diluted in a carrier oil).

CAUTIONS
May cause an allergic reaction in some individuals.

Carapa guianensis

COMMON NAMES Andiroba; bastard mahogany; carapa.
PLANT FAMILY Meliaceae.

RELATED SPECIES *C. granata* and *C. obovata* are also used medically.

RANGE Tropical America and Africa.

PARTS USED Bark, leaves, oil (from seeds).

OVERVIEW

Andiroba is a massive rainforest tree, reputed to be capable of growing up to 130m (420ft). The seed oil has a somewhat gruesome past having been used to preserve the severed heads of enemies by rainforest tribes. It is now finding a more positive lease of life as a popular medicinal oil. It relieves pain and inflammation, helps to heal wounds and clear rashes, and also acts as an excellent carrier oil for essential oils in aromatherapy massage.

PHYTOCHEMICALS

Oil Principally myristic and oleic acids.
Bark Alkaloid (andirobin).

ACTIONS

Analgesic, anti-inflammatory, antiparasitic, bitter, febrifuge, vermifuge.

INDICATIONS

Internally Fevers.
Externally Skin problems including parasite infestation, rashes, itching, psoriasis; arthritis and rheumatism.

PREPARATIONS

Internally Decoction of bark or leaves.
Externally Oil applied as a specific treatment or as a massage carrier oil. Leaves and bark applied or used as a bath.

CAUTIONS

None found.

Cassia occidentalis

COMMON NAMES Coffee senna; fedegoso; stinkweed.
PLANT FAMILY Leguminosae.

RELATED SPECIES There are over 500 *Cassia* species, many of which are medicinal. Not all are trees. The shrub *C. senna* is the source of the well-known laxative, senna pods. Other species include *C. alata*; *C. auriculata*; *C. fruticosa*; *C. grandis*; *C. ruiziana*; *C. tagera*.

NOT TO BE CONFUSED WITH *Cinnamomum cassia* (cassia bark). Confusingly, *Cassia* species are often referred to as *Senna* species instead.

RANGE *Cassia* species extend through tropical and warm temperate regions except for Europe. *C. occidentalis* is found in Africa and South America.

PARTS USED Flowers, fruits, leaves, roots, seeds.

OVERVIEW
While there are hundreds of *Cassia* species, *Cassia occidentalis* is representative of the group as a whole since it has a particularly wide range of uses. It is a small tree (up to 8m/25ft tall). Its seeds are used as a coffee substitute and are given in this form as a drink for asthma. Research has shown that leaf extracts protect the liver and are antibacterial. This tree has also shown anticancer properties in the laboratory.

PHYTOCHEMICALS
Leaves Flavonoid glycosides, anthraquinone pigments.
Roots Anthraquinones, apigenin, rhein.
Seeds Fatty acids, polysaccharides.

ACTIONS
Analgesic, anthelmintic, anti-inflammatory, antimicrobial, diuretic.

INDICATIONS
Internally
Flowers Bronchitis.
Leaves Abdominal pain, constipation, gout, hepatitis, period pain, snakebite and insect bites, syphilis, worm infestations especially roundworm.
Roots Fevers, malaria, period pain.
Seeds Asthma.
Externally
Leaves Skin problems including scabies.

PREPARATIONS
Internally All parts prepared by decoction. The leaves are used principally.
Externally Decoction.

CAUTIONS
Not to be used in pregnancy, reputed to cause abortions. Seeds may cause toxicity. To be taken on expert professional advice only.

Castanea sativa

COMMON NAME Spanish chestnut; sweet chestnut.
PLANT FAMILY Fagaceae.

RELATED SPECIES *C. dentata* (American chestnut); *C. pumila* (Allegheny chinkapin).

NOT TO BE CONFUSED WITH Sweet chestnut is not related to the horse chestnut (*Aesculus hippocastanum*).

RANGE Europe, the Mediterranean, North Africa.

PARTS USED Leaves, seeds (nuts).

OVERVIEW
The sweet chestnut is a long-lived and beautiful tree with distinctive long fronds of flowers. It can grow to around 30m (100ft) tall and sometimes up to 12m (40ft) in girth. Older trees will often lose their height, with branches and stem withering away, but continue to expand at the base of the trunk. The seeds (sweet chestnuts) themselves are edible nuts, encased in spiky shells. They are often served roasted. The leaves were once famed for their ability to relieve severe coughs including whooping cough but have now largely fallen out of use.

Flower remedy

Sweet chestnut is one of the Bach Flower Remedies, it is included in the category of remedies for 'despondency and despair' and is given 'for those moments which happen to some people when the anguish is so great as to seem to be unbearable'.

PHYTOCHEMICALS
Leaves Tannins.
Nuts Fatty acids, protein.

ACTIONS
Leaves Antitussive, astringent.
Nuts Nutritive.

INDICATIONS
Internally
Leaves Diarrhoea, heavy menstrual bleeding, rheumatism, spasmodic coughs, whooping cough.
Nuts Convalescence (as a nutritive food).
Externally
Leaves Pharyngitis.

PREPARATIONS
Internally
Leaves Decocted and taken by mouth.
Nuts Eaten.
Flowers Bach Flower Remedy.
Externally Decoction of leaves as a gargle for sore throats and pharyngitis.

CAUTIONS
None found.

Catha edulis

COMMON NAME Bushman's tea (English); khat (Arabic).
PLANT FAMILY Celastracae.

RANGE Africa.

PARTS USED Bark, leaves.

OVERVIEW
Khat is a small tree growing usually to 5m (15ft) but occasionally reaching up to twice this size. It is used in African and Arabian countries in a similar way to the coca bush (source of cocaine) in South America – the fresh leaves are chewed to improve strength and stamina and to lessen fatigue and hunger. The bark is boiled and used as a nerve tonic and stimulant to the heart. Concerns about problems of drug dependency with khat have led to its use being restricted in many countries.

PHYTOCHEMICALS
Flavonoids; phenethylamines (khatamines). The main phenethylamine (cathinone) has properties similar to amphetamine.

ACTIONS
Euphoric, stimulant. It also acts on the respiratory system.

INDICATIONS
Internally The leaves are traditionally used for fatigue and tiredness. Also for conditions of the chest including asthma and coughs.

PREPARATIONS
Internally The fresh leaves are chewed or the dried leaves are infused and drunk as a tea.

CAUTIONS
Use of the plant is restricted because it may cause dependency, although this is disputed. It has been suggested that khat may cause psychosis. It may also affect semen production.

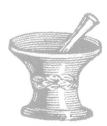

Cedrus atlantica

(sometimes considered a subspecies of *C. libani*, the cedar of Lebanon.)
COMMON NAME Atlantic cedar.
PLANT FAMILY Pinaceae.

NOT TO BE CONFUSED WITH Cedars are sometimes confused with members of the cypress family (*Cupressaceae*) because many of these use the word 'cedar' as part of their common names, such as *Thuja occidentalis* (eastern white cedar); *Thuja plicata* (western red cedar); *Juniperus virginiana* (red cedar). In aromatherapy the oil called 'cedarwood' is usually derived from *Juniperus virginiana*.

RANGE Africa to Asia.

PARTS USED Volatile oil, wood.

OVERVIEW

Cedars are evergreen trees in the pine family; they have needle leaves and produce cones. They can grow to a large size and have an impressive, stately appearance. Cedars have been widely planted as an ornamental tree (a blue variety is very popular). The oil they produce was used in embalming by the Egyptians. In aromatherapy it is applied to the scalp (mixed in a carrier oil) for dandruff and rubbed onto the chest for bronchitis. It is considered to break down deposits of fat in the skin and stimulate lymphatic drainage. Because of this, it has a reputation for treating cellulite.

Treatment tip – Cellulite

For cellulite you can try adding 3 or 4 drops of cedar oil to 10ml of sweet almond oil (or olive oil) and massaging this over areas of cellulite each morning and evening. Following a healthy low fat diet and doing regular exercise and skin brushing (to improve circulation) will also help to reduce cellulite.

PHYTOCHEMICALS

Volatile oil – mainly sesquiterpenes (cedrene), alcohols and ketones.

ACTIONS

Antiseptic, anticatarrhal, circulatory stimulant, expectorant.

INDICATIONS

Externally Chest infections, bronchitis, cellulite, chronic catarrh, dandruff, tuberculosis, impaired circulation, muscular aches and pains.

PREPARATIONS

Externally Steam inhalation for respiratory conditions. Application as a massage oil, diluted in a carrier oil, for poor circulation and muscle stiffness.

CAUTIONS

Avoid during pregnancy, may cause abortions.

Ceratonia siliqua

COMMON NAME Carob; locust bean; St John's bread.
PLANT FAMILY Leguminosae.

RANGE Arabia, Somalia.

PARTS USED Fruit (pod) and the seeds therein.

OVERVIEW

Carob is an evergreen tree whose pods are powdered and used as a non-stimulating alternative to chocolate.

It makes a good substitute for chocolate especially for hyperactive children and in migraines (which can often be triggered by eating chocolate). Chocolate addicts are also advised to try and wean themselves onto carob, as chocolate can exacerbate stress symptoms such as anxiety, shortness of breath and heart palpitations. As a medicine in its own right, carob is of primary value in treating diarrhoea; not only does it treat the symptoms of diarrhoea but it is also highly nutritious and helps to replace some of the nutrients lost during the illness. It has a key role in many of the regions where it grows because diarrhoea can still be a serious disease.

PHYTOCHEMICALS

Dietary fibre, polyphenols, tannins.

ACTIONS

Antidiarrhoeal, nutritive.

INDICATIONS

Internally In treatment of diarrhoea, especially if of acute onset; suitable for use in children. As an item of the diet to substitute chocolate in conditions such as hyperactivity in children, migraines and menstrual related food cravings.

PREPARATIONS

Internally Decoction of the roasted carob pod powder. Or carob pod juice. As a chocolate substitute it can be found as carob bars and other confections.

CAUTIONS

Carob is considered as a food and is generally safe and well tolerated.

Chionanthus virginicus

COMMON NAME Fringe tree; white fringetree; old man's beard.
PLANT FAMILY Oleaceae.

RELATED SPECIES *Fraxinus excelsior* (ash); *Olea europea* (olive).

NOT TO BE CONFUSED WITH *Clematis vitalba* (a climbing plant) is also known as old man's beard.

RANGE North America.

PART USED Bark (of roots and stem).

OVERVIEW

Fringe tree, a member of the olive family, is a small attractive tree with white flowers. It has a bitter tonic action, which means it is largely used to treat liver and gallbladder conditions. The Choctaw tribe used it externally to treat cuts, bruises and wounds. It was also formerly taken for malaria and typhoid fever. It is useful if you suffer from gallstones. Bitter liver and gallbladder stimulating herbs often give benefits in cases of migraines.

PHYTOCHEMICALS

Saponin (chionanthin), glycoside.

ACTIONS

Alterative, cholagogue, bitter tonic, hepatic, laxative.

Treatment tip – Gallbladder

If you suffer from gallbladder problems or recurrent migraines try taking 20 drops of Chionanthus tincture in water 1–3 times a day before meals. In migraines this may help to reduce the frequency of attacks (it is also important to make sure you are drinking enough fluids and to learn how to reduce and respond to stress).

INDICATIONS
Internally As a tonic convalescent aid to promote digestive functioning during recovery from illness; cirrhosis of the liver and chronic hepatitis; constipation; gallbladder disease; migraine; pancreatitis.
Externally Conjunctivitis, mouth ulcers and gum disease.

PREPARATIONS
Internally Decoction or tincture.
Externally Decoction taken as an eye bath for conjunctivitis, or as a mouthwash for mouth and gum disease.

CAUTIONS
None found.

Cinchona species

COMMON NAME Cinchona; Peruvian bark; Jesuit's bark.
PLANT FAMILY Rubiaceae.

RELATED SPECIES It is difficult to tell the various *Cinchona* species apart. The principal species used are *C. calisaya*; *C. ledgeriana*; *C. pubescens*; *C. succirubra*.

RANGE Tropical America – Andes to Costa Rica. Cultivated widely elsewhere including India.

PART USED Bark.

OVERVIEW
Historically this is one of the most important and widely used of all medicinal trees. *Cinchona* species are evergreen South American trees yielding the anti-malarial alkaloid quinine. The discovery of quinine made Cinchona trees in high demand and huge efforts were made to secure supplies of this seemingly miraculous drug. Although the importance of quinine has declined since being super-seded by synthetic drugs, it is undergoing a renaissance as many of the newer

drugs are developing problems with resistance. Another alkaloid, quinidine, is used in conventional medicine to treat irregular heartbeat (arythmias). Quinine continues to be a constituent of tonic water to which it imparts a bitter, astringent flavour. *Cinchona* is famous in homeopathy as being one of the first substances tested by its founder Samuel Hahnemann.

PHYTOCHEMICALS
Quinoline alkaloids (principally quinine, also quinidine), glycosides, tannin, resin.

ACTIONS
Antimalarial, antispasmodic, astringent, bitter, febrifuge.

INDICATIONS
Internally Colds and influenza, fevers, irregular heartbeats, malaria, muscle cramps.

PREPARATIONS
Internally Tincture or decoction of the bark.

CAUTIONS
Cinchona is subject to restrictions in some countries. It should only be taken on expert professional advice. A syndrome called cinchonism can develop with headaches, abdominal pain and aural and visual disturbances. It is potentially damaging to the nervous system and can cause deafness. Avoid in pregnancy. It should not be used in conjunction with certain conventional drugs such as heart and ulcer medicines and antihistamines.

Cinnamomum zeylanicum

(also known as *C. verum*)
COMMON NAME Cinnamon.
PLANT FAMILY Lauaraceae.

RELATED SPECIES *C. camphora* (camphor tree) – this large evergreen tree is a source of camphor oil, a volatile oil used for arthritis and chest infections. *C. cassia* (also known as *C. aromaticum*) is a Chinese species sometimes used in place of *C. zeylanicum* but it is considered inferior.

RANGE South-west India, Sri Lanka.

PARTS USED Bark; essential oil distilled from bark or leaf.

OVERVIEW

The bark of the cinnamon tree is a famous spice and scent. It is mentioned in the Bible in Exodus 31: 'The Lord spake unto Moses to make an oil of holy anointment of myrrh, cinnamon, cassia and olive oil. He was directed to anoint the area of prayer and all its contents... And thou shalt sanctify them, that they may be most holy'. Its remarkable taste and smell make it a popular flavouring, especially for sweet foods. It is also used in toothpaste and as an incense. The main constituent is the volatile oil, which has antiseptic and pain-relieving properties. The bark has a warming and relaxing effect on the digestive system and is pleasantly warming to the circulation as a whole. It has a particular role to play in treating a variety of digestive disorders and in various infections. A decoction of the bark (cinnamon quills) makes a very pleasant digestive tea that can be taken on a regular basis. Cinnamon bark tincture has been shown to inhibit *Helicobacter pylori* (the organism that causes many cases of stomach and duodenal ulcers). The tea is wonderful for indigestion and flatulence and can relieve headaches. When you drink cinnamon tea savour the aroma as the scent will also help to calm and relax you. An easy and delightful way to enjoy cinnamon is as cinnamon toast – simply make toast, spread on margarine and a little brown sugar then sprinkle on cinnamon powder.

Treatment tip – Period pain

You can take cinnamon tincture or tea for period pain; it eases muscle spasms reducing the pain. Take 2–5ml of the tincture in warm water up to 4 times a day for this problem, or drink hot cinnamon tea.

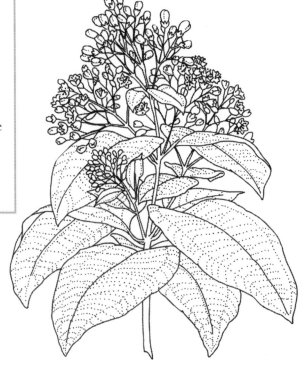

PHYTOCHEMICALS
Volatile oil (principally cinnamic aldehyde in the bark and eugenol in the leaf); tannins.

ACTIONS
Analgesic, antibacterial, antifungal, antiviral, antispasmodic, aromatic bitter, carminative, circulatory stimulant, expectorant.

INDICATIONS
Internally candidiasis, colds and influenza, coughs and chest infections, indigestion, flatulence, headaches, high blood pressure, nausea, period pain, stomach and muscle aches and cramps; gastric and duodenal ulcers; also used in convalescence to support the digestion and aid recovery.
Externally Bacterial and fungal skin infections, coughs and colds, muscular stiffness.

PREPARATIONS
Internally Decoction and tincture.
Externally Steam inhalation for coughs and colds. Massage rub diluted in a carrier oil for infections and muscular spasms.

CAUTIONS
The volatile oil causes skin irritation in some people.

Citrus aurantium

COMMON NAME Bitter orange; neroli; bigarade.
PLANT FAMILY Rutaceae.

RELATED SPECIES *C. aurantiifolia* (lime); *C. limon* (lemon); *C.* x *paradisi* (grapefruit); *C. reticulata* (mandarin orange).

RANGE South-east Asia.

PARTS USED Volatile oil distilled from the flowers, leaves or peel; fruit; leaves.

Treatment tip – Low mood

If you are prone to dips in your mood you could try carrying a little bottle of neroli with you to inhale when you feel low. If you have difficulty sleeping, one or two drops in a little almond oil makes a good massage oil to be applied on going to bed.

OVERVIEW

The *Citrus* species are enormously complex in terms of the medicinal products they can yield. None more so than bitter orange. The essential oils are particularly confounding! The oil from the leaves is called 'petitgrain bigarade', that from the flowers is 'neroli bigarade', and from the peel is 'orange bigarade'. Neroli is the most prized (and the most expensive) and is famed for its effects on improving the mood and treating various psychological disorders. It is also useful on the physical level, particularly as an antiseptic. A recent study showed that the fruit inhibits rotavirus, which causes diarrhoea.

PHYTOCHEMICALS

Coumarins; volatile oil (composition varies depending on the part of the plant it is harvested from); flavonoids; vitamin C. Neroli oil contains hydrocarbons (pinenes and limonene), alcohols (especially linalool), and esters (linalyl acetate).

ACTIONS

Fruit and peel Anti-inflammatory, antiseptic, immunostimulant, nutritive.
Neroli oil Antibacterial, nervous trophorestorative, sedative.

INDICATIONS

Internally Convalescence, poor digestion, flatulence.
Externally Anxiety, depression, insomnia.

PREPARATIONS

Internally
Fruit Eaten fresh.
Peel Infusion.
Externally
Volatile oil Inhalation or as a massage oil diluted in a carrier oil.
Flower water A mild relaxant and sedative. (Buy carefully, as most commercially available flower waters are merely synthetically fragranced products.)

CAUTIONS

Avoid undiluted volatile oils coming into direct contact with the skin. Wash your hands after handling volatile oils.

Citrus limon

COMMON NAME Lemon.
PLANT FAMILY Rutaceae.

RELATED SPECIES See *C. aurantium*.

RANGE South-east Asia.

PARTS USED Fruit (juice and peel); volatile oil (distilled from the fruit peel).

OVERVIEW

This evergreen fruit tree has a number of medicinal uses. Lemons are rich in bioflavanoids, which help to strengthen the circulation and heal varicose veins. They can reduce or prevent arteriosclerosis and are therefore helpful in decreasing the risk of heart disease. Lemon juice also stimulates the digestion and is an immune booster. A glassful of lemon juice a day (1–2 lemons squeezed, mixed with other juices to offset the sharpness) is a wonderfully healthy and refreshing addition to the diet. Lemons are often given in drinks for cold and influenza.

PHYTOCHEMICALS

Bioflavanoids, vitamins A, B and C, volatile oil (principally limonene).

ACTIONS

Anti-inflammatory, antioxidant, antiseptic, immunostimulant, nutritive.

Treatment tip – Colds and flu

A good warming and immune enhancing drink for colds and flu, or just as a general comforter on cold days, is made as follows. Mix together the juice of 1–2 lemons, 2–4 teaspoons of elderflower cordial and a couple of slivers of crushed fresh ginger; pour on boiling water, cover with a saucer for 5 minutes then stir and drink. Delicious!

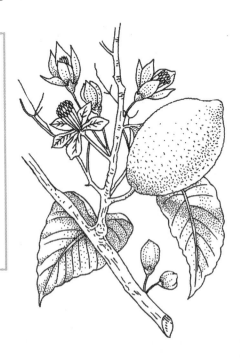

INDICATIONS
Internally Arteriosclerosis, conditions causing easy bruising, haemorrhoids, supportive treatment in infections and during convalescence, varicose veins.
Externally
Fruit Insect bite and stings, sore throats.
Volatile oil Boils, headaches, insect bites and stings, insomnia, nausea.

PREPARATIONS
Internally freshly squeezed fruit juice taken by mouth.
Externally
Fruit Cut in half and applied directly to bites and stings as a domestic emergency treatment. The juice as a gargle for sore throats.
Volatile oil As an inhalation or applied as a massage oil diluted in a carrier oil.

CAUTIONS
Avoid undiluted volatile oils coming into direct contact with the skin. Wash your hands after handling volatile oils.

Cola nitida

COMMON NAME Cola; kola.
PLANT FAMILY Sterculiaceae.

RELATED SPECIES *C. acuminata*; *C. anomala*; *C. greenwayi*; *C. verticillata*.

RANGE Africa.

PART USED Seeds (cola nuts).

OVERVIEW
Cola nuts are chewed to relieve fatigue and depress hunger. Essentially they have a stimulating effect on the body due to the presence of caffeine (and another stimulant, theobromine). A drink was prepared for hard-working frontiers people in North America to help them cope with the demands of their tough life. This combined cola nuts with another plant renowned for improving stamina – the leaves of the coca bush (source of cocaine). It was called coca-cola. Cola nuts may seem to offer help in dealing with the demands of modern life but, in fact, the initial energy stimulation given by caffeine is followed by a depressant effect.

PHYTOCHEMICALS
Caffeine (2.5%), phenolics, tannins, theobromine.

ACTIONS

Bitter, diuretic, stimulant (to heart and respiration).

INDICATIONS

Internally To relieve fatigue; stimulation of digestion.

PREPARATIONS

Internally The nuts are chewed. A tincture is available.

CAUTIONS

Cola should not be taken if you suffer from anxiety, headaches, high blood pressure or hyperactivity as it can exacerbate these conditions. Chewing of the nuts is not advised as it has been suggested that this may play a role in causing cancer.

Commiphora molmol

(also known as C. myrrha)
COMMON NAME Myrrh.
PLANT FAMILY Burseraceae.

RELATED SPECIES *C. africana* (hairy corkwood); *C. gileadensis* (balm of Gilead); *C. wightii* (guggul).

RANGE North-east Africa to Arabia.

PART USED Oleo-gum resin exuded from the bark.

OVERVIEW

This small deciduous tree is the source of the Biblical myrrh. Myrrh is an oleo-gum resin, a gelatinous substance produced by the bark, which sets hard when drying. It was used by the Egyptians for embalming. Myrrh is highly antiseptic and is useful for a number of different infections of the skin and mouth. It is excellent for treating thrush (*candida*) in the mouth and dental abscesses. You can use myrrh cream for any pustular spots and boils and mix the tincture with warm water to make an excellent gargle that is effective in treating sore throats.

PHYTOCHEMICALS
Gums, resins, volatile oil.

ACTIONS
Antiseptic, astringent, local circulatory stimulant, immunostimulant.

INDICATIONS
Externally Acne, boils, fungal skin infections (athlete's foot, ringworm, scabies), oral and vaginal thrush. Mouth and gum infections generally, dental abscesses, tonsillitis and throat infections.

PREPARATIONS
Externally Resins are not water soluble so the most useful myrrh preparation is a tincture made with alcohol at a strength of 96%. This should be used well diluted with water. It can be used as a gargle for tonsillitis, as a mouthwash for thrush and other oral infections, as a cream for skin infections and as a douche for vaginal thrush.

CAUTIONS
Myrrh resin is corrosive to the skin and should not be used neat, especially in tincture form. It is generally only used externally. Swallowing may cause stomach irritation.

Commiphora wightii

(also known as *Commiphora mukul*)
COMMON NAME Guggul.
PLANT FAMILY Burseraceae.

RELATED SPECIES see *C. molmol*.

RANGE Arabia, India.

PART USED Oleo-gum resin exuded from the bark.

OVERVIEW
Guggul is a small thorny tree with peeling bark that has stimulated a lot of interest in recent years due to its ability to assist in lowering cholesterol levels. This can result in reducing the risk of heart disease. Traditionally it has been used in Ayurvedic medicine for obesity and this could be due to its effects on lowering the level of harmful fats in the body. A standardized extract known as gugulipid is available which offers a genuine safe and effective alternative to conventional cholesterol lowering drugs.

PHYTOCHEMICALS
Gum, resin, volatile oil. Steroids (guggulsterones).

ACTIONS
Anti-inflammatory, antioxidant, antiseptic, hypocholesterolaemic.

INDICATIONS
Internally Acne, rheumatoid arthritis, high cholesterol levels.

PREPARATIONS
Internally Tincture or standardized extract.

CAUTIONS
Tinctures and crude oleo-gum resin can cause skin rashes and diarrhoea. The standardized extract appears to be better tolerated and is therefore the preparation of choice. Guggul should be avoided when breastfeeding.

Cornus species

COMMON NAMES See under Related Species.
Collectively *Cornus* trees are known as 'dogwoods'.
PLANT FAMILY Cornaceae.

RELATED SPECIES Among the many species used are *C. alternatifolia* (alternate leaf dogwood); *C. canadensis* (Bunchberry dogwood); *C. florida* (American boxwood); *C. mas* (cornelian cherry); *C. nuttallii* (Pacific dogwood); *C. officinalis* (shan zhu yu); *C. sanguinea* (swamp dogwood); *C. sericea* (Red osier dogwood).

RANGE Cornus species occur in Africa, Asia, Europe, North and South America.

PARTS USED Fruits, root and stem bark (*C. florida*); fruits (*C. officinalis*).

OVERVIEW
Dogwood trees (some species are shrubs) have been used as medicines throughout the world, especially in China and North America. Many species are grown

as ornamentals on account of their beautiful foliage and striking bracts (leaf-like structures underlying the flowers that actually look more like large petals). *Cornus florida*, a North American species, was formerly used as a substitute for Cinchona in treating malarial fevers and was applied to the skin to treat anthrax sores. *Cornus officinalis* is used in traditional Chinese medicine as a remedy to 'stabilize and bind'. It tones the kidneys and liver, and reduces heavy menstrual bleeding.

PHYTOCHEMICALS
C. florida – Betulic and gallic acids, gum, iridoid glycoside (verbenalin), resin, tannins.
C. officinalis – Tannins, saponins, ursolic acid, verbenalin.

ACTIONS
C. florida – Anthelmintic, antiseptic, astringent, febrifuge, tonic.
C. officinalis – Astringent, diuretic, hepatic, possible hypotensive.

INDICATIONS
Internally
C. florida – Backache associated with pregnancy, fatigue, fevers, diarrhoea, digestive disorders, headaches.
C. officinalis – Excessive sweating, heavy menstrual bleeding, incontinence of urine, possibly for high blood pressure, premature ejaculation.
Externally
C. florida – Skin ulcers.

PREPARATIONS
Internally Both species prepared by decoction. *C. florida* bark was chewed for headaches.
Externally Decoction of *C. florida*.

CAUTIONS
Cornus officinalis should not be taken when it is painful or difficult to pass urine.

Corylus avellana

COMMON NAMES European hazel; filbert.
PLANT FAMILY Betulaceae.

RELATED SPECIES *C. americana* (American hazelnut); *C. cornuta* (beaked hazelnut) and its varieties.

RANGE Eurasia.

PARTS USED Leaves, nuts, nut oil.

OVERVIEW
Hazel is a small tree often planted in hedgerows or coppiced (cut back to the ground to stimulate re-growth) for fuel and fencing materials. Hazel produces long, straight, flexible shoots (hazel wands) long used for divination of water. The nuts are highly nutritious and widely used. A group of constituents called oligomeric proanthocyanidins can be extracted from the leaves. These support collagen in the body's connective tissues and can be useful in treating varicose veins and bruising. The fresh nuts of American hazelnut were taken by Iroquois women to give them strength during pregnancy. Hazelnut oil has a pleasantly nutty aroma and taste. It is a good nourishing oil for promoting healthy skin and hair. Try using it in salad dressings and as an alternative to butter or margarine to spread on bread. Recent research has revealed that hazel leaves contain the anti-cancer compound taxol.

PHYTOCHEMICALS
Leaves Flavonols (oligomeric proanthocyanidins).

ACTIONS
Leaves – Astringent, vulnerary.
Nuts – Nutritive.

INDICATIONS
Internally
Leaves Diarrhoea, bruising and varicose veins.
Nuts Nutritive in convalescence.
Internally and Externally
Hazelnut oil To improve the skin and hair.

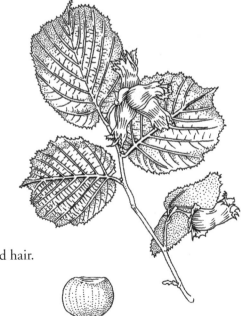

PREPARATIONS
Internally
Leaves Decoction for diarrhoea. Leaf extract taken for varicose veins.
Nuts Eaten.
Hazelnut oil Used as part of the diet or applied externally to skin and hair.

CAUTIONS
None found.

Crataegus species

COMMON NAMES Hawthorn; May tree.
PLANT FAMILY Rosaceae.

RELATED SPECIES *C. laevigata* and *C. monogyna* frequently hybridize with each other so that many hawthorns cannot be identified as being definitely one or the other. Several North American species have medicinal properties including *C. chrysocarpa* (fireberry hawthorn); *C. douglasii* (black hawthorn); *C. pinnatifida* (Chinese hawthorn).

RANGE Northern temperate region.

PARTS USED Flowers, fruits, leaves.

OVERVIEW
Hawthorn is one of the most important trees in European herbal medicine. It is a twisted and thorny tree often grown in hedges, with bright red fruits known as hawthorn berries or haws. In England it tends to begin flowering at the beginning of May hence the common name of May tree. It is known as 'the father of the heart' and is used to treat a variety of heart and circulatory problems. The flowers, fruits and leaves contain potent chemical

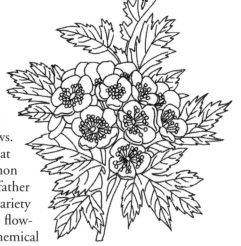

compounds that act as antioxidants to protect the heart's tissues from damage. Hawthorn preparations relax the blood vessels that supply the heart (coronary arteries), and this improves the blood supply to the heart and relieves angina. They also strengthen the beating of the heart, making it more efficient; this is very useful in cases of heart failure. Its actions can help to lower the blood pressure. The great value of hawthorn is that, although it can have profound healing effects, it achieves these in a gentle and supportive way. The tea made from the leaves and flowers is pleasant and can be taken on a daily basis to help protect the heart and circulation.

PHYTOCHEMICALS

Flavonoids (including quercetin glycosides: – hyperoside, rutin); oligomeric procyanidins.

ACTIONS

Antiarrythmic, antioxidant, astringent (mild), cardiac trophorestorative, hypotensive, stabilizes collagen.

INDICATIONS

Internally Angina, atherosclerosis, congestive heart failure and its symptoms (shortness of breath, swelling of ankles, chest pain), heart arrythmias, high blood pressure, peripheral arterial disease.
Externally Sore throats.

PREPARATIONS

Internally
Flowers and leaves 2–4g a day by infusion or decoction.
Berries 2–4g a day by decoction.
Flowers, leaves and berries Tincture, 1:5, 45% alcohol. Take 3–15 ml/day in water.
Externally The decoction is used as a gargle for sore throats.

CAUTIONS

Hawthorn is generally considered safe and well tolerated. However it does have an effect on angiotensin-converting enzyme which is involved in the regulation of blood pressure, so it probably should not be given alongside conventional drugs that also act on this mechanism (ACE inhibitors or other blood pressure lowering drugs). People with low blood pressure should avoid hawthorn as it may lower the pressure still further.

Crataeva nurvala

COMMON NAMES Varuna; three-leaved caper.
PLANT FAMILY Capparidaceae.

RELATED SPECIES *C. benthamii; C. tapia.*

RANGE India

PARTS USED Stem and root bark.

OVERVIEW

A deciduous tree, *Crataeva nurvala* is one of the main Ayurvedic medicines for the urinary system. It has been used in India for at least 3,000 years. It is used for urinary tract infections, to strengthen the bladder wall and prevent and treat bladder and kidney stones. It helps to improve the symptoms of prostate disease in men, such as weak flow of urine.

PHYTOCHEMICALS
Flavonoids, glucosinolates, saponins, sterols, tannins.

ACTIONS
Anti-inflammatory, antilithic, urinary trophorestorative.

INDICATIONS
Internally Benign prostatic hypertrophy, bladder and kidney stones, cystitis, incontinence of urine.

PREPARATIONS
Internally Decoctions or tincture of the stem or root bark.

CAUTIONS
None found.

Crescentia cujete

COMMON NAME Calabash tree.
PLANT FAMILY Bignoniaceae.

RANGE Tropical America.

PARTS USED Fruit, leaves.

OVERVIEW
The most distinctive feature of this small tree is its huge round green fruits, weighing up to 10kg (22lbs). The fruits are hollowed out and used as gourds. The pith lining the fruits is used to treat a variety of chest conditions including asthma. The leaves are used medicinally for toothache. Studies have shown the leaves and stem bark to be effective against a broad range of infections.

PHYTOCHEMICALS
Unclear.

ACTIONS
Antibacterial (bark and leaves); emmenagogue, pectoral (fruit).

INDICATIONS
Internally Asthma, bronchitis, coughs.

PREPARATIONS
Internally The fruit pith is decocted. The leaves are chewed for toothache.

CAUTIONS
Internal use is not advised unless under expert professional advice. Avoid in pregnancy as it may cause abortion.

Croton eleuteria

COMMON NAME Cascarilla.
PLANT FAMILY Euphorbiaceae.

RELATED SPECIES Many *Croton* species are used medicinally including *C. cuneatus*; *C. glabellus*; *C. gratissimus*; *C. lechleri*; *C. malambo*; *C. palanostigma*; *C. tiglium*; *C. trinitatis*.

RANGE West Indies.

PARTS USED Bark, leaves.

OVERVIEW
Cascarilla is a small tree and the source of cascarilla bark. This is used to treat a range of digestive problems and fevers. A number of other Croton trees are used as medicines. *C. tiglium* is the source of croton oil (extracted from the seeds), which is one of the most drastically purgative substances known. It has been used as a treatment of last resort for severe constipation but should not be used as a medicine because it is carcinogenic and highly toxic. *C. lechleri* is commonly known as dragon's blood after the red resin secreted from its bark. The resin is also a drastic purgative like croton oil, however its sap has traditionally been used for cancer and tuberculosis and it is currently being researched to try and develop conventional drugs for these diseases.

PHYTOCHEMICALS
Bitter; tannins; volatile oil.

ACTIONS
Aromatic; bitter tonic; expectorant.

INDICATIONS
Internally Chronic bronchitis; digestive disorders including diarrhoea, dysentery, flatulence, indigestion; fevers.

PREPARATIONS
Internally Bark and leaves are taken as a decoction. The bark is used more widely than the leaves.

CAUTIONS
None found.

Cupressus sempervirens

COMMON NAMES Cypress; Italian cypress.
PLANT FAMILY Cupressaceae.

RANGE Southern Europe.

PARTS USED Volatile oil distilled from the leaves or cones.

Conservation

C. sempervirens is widely planted throughout the Mediterranean and is not endangered. It is however classed as being vulnerable to extinction in the wild in Turkey and northern Iran.

OVERVIEW
Cypress trees are evergreen conifers. In the wild the Italian cypress has horizontal branches (*C. sempervirens* var. *horizontalis*) but it is most commonly grown as a variety with vertical branches. This columnar structure makes the tree look like an elegant needle which, when skilfully planted, gives a striking vertical relief to the landscape. It is characteristic of Italy and the Mediterranean as a whole. Its main contribution to medicine is its volatile oil. This is used particularly to treat respiratory disorders, such as chest infections, and circulatory problems. Applied to the legs, diluted in a carrier oil, it is particularly helpful for varicose veins. Try adding 2 drops of the volatile oil to 10ml of sweet almond oil and massaging gently over varicose veins each morning and evening. The tree contains chemicals called oligomeric procyanidins, which are noted for their protective effects on the heart and circulation.

PHYTOCHEMICALS
Oligomeric procyanidins; volatile oil – monoterpenes (especially an α-pinene), alcohols, oxides, esters.

ACTIONS
Antibacterial, antispasmodic, antitussive, astringent.

INDICATIONS

Externally

Respiratory system – bronchitis, chest infections, whooping cough.
Circulatory system – broken capillaries, haemorrhoids, varicose veins.

PREPARATIONS

Externally As an inhalation and chest rub (diluted in a carrier oil) for chest problems. Applied to the skin (diluted in a carrier oil) for circulatory problems.

CAUTIONS

Avoid undiluted volatile oils coming into direct contact with the skin. Wash your hands after handling volatile oils.

Cydonia oblonga

COMMON NAME Quince.
PLANT FAMILY Rosaceae.

RELATED SPECIES *Chaenomeles speciosa* (japonica; Japanese quince).

RANGE Western Asia.

PARTS USED Fruit, seeds.

OVERVIEW

The quince is a small tree that has long been grown for its aromatic edible fruit. The quince fruit can be made into a jelly or marmalade and is used as an ingredient in various sweet dishes. When grown in warm climates the fruit can be eaten raw. There is much folklore attached to this tree; it was thought to protect against evil influences, and is referred to in numerous texts from the Bible to Virgil. It was long seen as a symbol of love and was eaten by newlyweds at marriage celebrations. You might consider planting a quince in your garden, ideally outside your front door as this is said to bring love and happiness and to protect the home! Medicinally the fruit provides important nutritive elements and is an excellent food to take to help treat fatigue, debility and aid recovery from illness. The seeds are rich in mucilage, a gelatinous substance that acts as a bulk-forming laxative (much like the better known linseeds) and is soothing to various inflammatory problems in the digestive system. It was also formerly used to soothe irritation felt in the urinary tract when passing water.

PHYTOCHEMICALS
Fruits Tannins, vitamin C.
Seeds Amygdalin, fixed oil, mucilage.

ACTIONS
Fruits Astringent, nutritive.
Seeds Anti-inflammatory, demulcent, laxative.

INDICATIONS
Internally
Fruits An aid to recovery in convalescence; diarrhoea, dysentery.
Seeds Constipation, dry irritable coughs, inflammatory digestive disorders.
Externally
Seeds Burns, dry skin, inflammatory mouth problems.

PREPARATIONS
Internally
Fruit Eaten raw or cooked, in convalescence and as a dietary aid.
Seeds Decoction or infusion.
Externally
Seeds Infused or decocted to release mucilage and taken as a mouthwash for sore oral conditions, applied as a poultice or incorporated into creams and lotions for burns and dry skin.

CAUTIONS
None found.

Ekebergia capensis

COMMON NAMES Cape ash, dog plum (English); umnyamathi (Zulu).
PLANT FAMILY Meliaceae.

RANGE South Africa.

PARTS USED The bark principally, but also leaves and roots.

OVERVIEW
Cape ash is a medium-sized (growing up to 12m/40ft) rough barked African tree. It has been little researched and not much is known about its constituents. It is used by native tribes to treat a wide range of problems including skin diseases, and digestive and chest disorders. The tree is seen as a sacred plant offering protection from evil and is also used as a love charm. (This might connect with the traditional use of the bark to treat infertility.) It has recently shown promise in tests to find plants that are active against tuberculosis.

PHYTOCHEMICALS
Unclear.

ACTIONS
Astringent, emetic, purgative.

INDICATIONS
Internally Traditionally used for dysentery, heartburn, infertility (bark); parasite infestation, headaches (leaves); cough, gastritis, headache.
Externally Abscesses, acne, boils (bark); scabies (roots).

PREPARATIONS
Internally/Externally Decoctions of powdered bark or root. Taken by mouth or applied externally to skin disorders.

CAUTIONS
Cape ash preparations may cause vomiting and diarrhoea.

Erythrina lysistemon

COMMON NAMES Common coral tree (English); umsinsi (Zulu).
PLANT FAMILY Leguminosae.

RELATED SPECIES *E. abyssinica, E. burana, E. caffra, E. latissima, E. sigmoidea.*

RANGE Africa.

PARTS USED The bark principally, but also the leaves and roots.

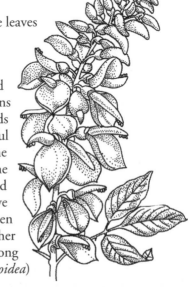

OVERVIEW
This handsome tree with delightful bright red flowers is widely cultivated in parks and gardens as an ornamental tree. Despite its beauty it needs to be treated carefully as it contains powerful alkaloids that can have strong effects on the body. It is used to relieve the pain of toothache and earache and to treat skin infections and wounds. Strips of the bark are used by native tribes to tie up bundles of herbs, which are then boiled to make a tea to facilitate childbirth. Other *Erythrina* species have been shown to have strong relaxant effects on the digestive system (*E. sigmoidea*) and to be antimicrobial (*E. abyssinica*).

PHYTOCHEMICALS
Alkaloids (present in most parts of the tree), isoflavonoids, glycosides.

ACTIONS
Analgesic, antibacterial, anti-inflammatory.

INDICATIONS
Internally Traditionally used for arthritis, and toothache.
Externally Abscesses, earache, sores and wounds.

PREPARATIONS
Internally Decoction of the bark.
Externally Poultice of the bark for abscesses, sores and wounds. Infusion of the leaves used as ear drops for earache.

CAUTIONS
Erythrina species contain potentially toxic alkaloids, they should only be used on expert professional advice.

Erythrophleum lasianthum

COMMON NAMES Swazi ordeal tree, red water tree (English);
umbhemise (Zulu).
PLANT FAMILY Leguminosae.

RELATED SPECIES *E. suaveolens.*

NOT TO BE CONFUSED WITH The ordeal bean of Calabar (*Physostigma venenosum*).

RANGE South Africa.

PARTS USED Principally the bark. The seeds are less frequently used due to having a higher degree of toxicity.

OVERVIEW
The Swazi ordeal tree is so called because of the poisonous nature of its alkaloids and their use in native African justice systems. A person found guilty of a serious crime might be given a preparation of this tree, or one of the other ordeal plants, and then observed to see what happens. If they survive they are seen as innocent, if they die then guilt is proven beyond doubt. This system may sound somewhat less than infallible but native people believed that the tree had the power to divine a person's guilt and to mete out punishment if necessary. Despite its inherent dangers it has been used to treat spasmodic and painful conditions. Some *Erythrophleum* species have been shown to lower blood pressure.

PHYTOCHEMICALS
Alkaloids (including cassaine and erythrophleine).

ACTIONS
Analgesic, antispasmodic.

INDICATIONS
Internally Traditionally used for digestive spasms, fevers, and for treating pain (general pain anywhere in the body, and headaches, migraine).

PREPARATIONS
Internally Decoctions of the bark are drunk or the powdered bark is taken as a snuff or licked from the hand.

CAUTIONS
This plant is potentially toxic and should only be taken on expert professional advice.

Eucalyptus globulus

COMMON NAMES Blue gum, Tasmanian blue gum, fever tree.
PLANT FAMILY Myrtaceae.

RELATED SPECIES There are at least 450 different *Eucalyptus* species, many of which have medicinal properties including *E. citriodora* (lemon scented gum); *E. dives* (peppermint gum); *E. polybractea* (silver malee scrub); *E. radiata* (white top peppermint); *E. smithii* (gully gum); *E. staigeriana* (lemon-scented iron bark).

RANGE Native to Australia, grown in many other countries.

PARTS USED Bark, leaves and the volatile oil distilled from the leaves, oleo-resin (kino).

Treatment tip – Insomnia

E. staigeriana is great for insomnia. Just before going to bed take a warm bath and then either have someone massage the oil onto your back and feet or use the oil as a room fragrance. This often helps to promote a good night's sleep.

OVERVIEW
The fast growing, evergreen *Eucalyptus* trees are synonymous with the Australian countryside. There are numerous species appearing in many different sizes (some

species are amongst the tallest trees in the world while others are small shrubs) and colours. A recent novel has created a modern fable about a *Eucalyptus* tree collector who set his daughter's suitors the task of identifying every species of Eucalyptus before giving her hand in marriage. Classification of *Eucalypti* is complex but they are generally divided into 6 groups based on their bark characteristics – bloodwoods, boxes, gums, ironbarks, peppermints and stringybarks. Rich in volatile oils they are commonly fragrant, and their peeling barks offer an appealing variety of shades and textures. The volatile oils are the main medicinal substances in the trees and their usefulness and diversity make them particularly important in aromatherapy and aromatic medicine. Some species yield an oleo-resin known as kino. *Eucalyptus globulus*, blue gum, is the most frequently cultivated species of *Eucalyptus* and is also the most commonly used medicinal species. Its volatile oil has the distinctive aromatic 'disinfectant' *Eucalyptus* smell, other species smell strongly of lemon or peppermint. It has valuable effects on the respiratory system helping to kill off infection, open up the airways and reduce congestion. It is good to keep a bottle of the oil on hand and use it as an inhalation for coughs and colds. *E. globulus* oil is sometimes too irritating to the airways to use in small children and sensitive adults. In these cases *E. smithii* can be used instead. The volatile oil of this species is so mild that it can often be used as a massage oil without the need to be diluted in a carrier oil. *E. staigeriana* has a wonderful soft lemon scent that is relaxing and sedative. It can be applied as a massage oil (diluted in a carrier oil) for the effects of tension and stress on the muscles.

PHYTOCHEMICALS
Leaves Flavonoids (including hyperoside and rutin); polyphenolic acids; volatile oil.
The volatile oil itself contains mostly (up to 85%) 1,8-cineole (eucalyptol).

ACTIONS
Antiseptic, antispasmodic, circulatory stimulant, decongestant, expectorant, febrifuge.

INDICATIONS
Externally Abscesses, catarrh, bronchitis, coughs (especially productive coughs), emphysema, fevers, muscular spasms, sprains. Used as an inhalation for nasal congestion and sinusitis.

PREPARATIONS
Externally The leaves can be decocted or infused and used as an inhalation. The volatile oil is used as an inhalation and as a rub (diluted in a massage carrier oil).

CAUTIONS
Eucalyptus globulus can be too irritating to the respiratory system of young children or sensitive adults. Use with caution in asthmatics, it may make symptoms

worse. Avoid undiluted volatile oils coming into direct contact with the skin. Wash you hands after handling volatile oils.

Euonymus species

COMMON NAME See under Species Used.
PLANT FAMILY Celastraceae.

SPECIES USED spindle tree, wahoo, Indian arrow wood (*E. atropurpurea*); spindle tree (*E. purpurea*).

RANGE North America (*E. atropurpurea*); Europe, Western Asia (*E. purpurea*).

PARTS USED Bark principally but also the roots and berries.

OVERVIEW
The spindle tree gains its name from the use of its wood to make spindles for weaving. The American and European species are used in similar ways although *E. atropurpurea* is used more commonly. Both species are small deciduous trees with striking brightly-coloured fruits. The fruits of *E. atropurpurea* are purple with red seeds. The fruits of *E. purpurea* range from pink to orange to red, all in vivid shades, opening to reveal luminous orange seeds. The leaves also provide delightful colour changes in autumn. Frequently planted as a hedgerow tree in the UK, it lights up the field boundaries and roadsides on dull autumn days. Spindle tree bark stimulates the gall bladder and liver and has a laxative effect. The American Eclectic doctors used it for liver enlargement and as a tonic to help patients recover from malaria. If you have the right space though you might want to plant one or more of these trees to enjoy the sight of their strange and wonderful fruits!

PHYTOCHEMICALS
E. atropurpurea – cardenolide glycosides, sterols, tannins.

ACTIONS
Anthelmintic, appetite stimulant, cholagogue, depurative, laxative.

INDICATIONS
Internally Constipation, skin disorders such as acne and psoriasis, worm infestation (children and adults).

PREPARATIONS
Internally Bark as a decoction or tincture.

CAUTIONS

The berries can cause diarrhoea and vomiting. The dosage of all parts of the spindle tree must be carefully calculated to avoid causing digestive upsets, and so it should only be taken on expert professional advice. It should not be taken during pregnancy.

Fagus sylvatica

COMMON NAME Beech.
PLANT FAMILY Fagaceae.

RELATED SPECIES Several cultivars of beech are planted ornamentally including copper beech and weeping beech but these are not used medicinally. *F. grandifolia*, the American beech, was used medically by native tribes in several ways including chewing the nuts for worm infestations (Cherokee).

RANGE Europe.

PARTS USED Nut oil, tar from the wood.

OVERVIEW

The beech tree is large (40m/140ft in height) majestic and impressive. The trunk and branches are muscular, almost like huge animal limbs in appearance, the silver grey bark is like elephant hide. Its wood is used for a variety of purposes including making furniture, parquet floors and as an excellent source of fuel. The timber was once used as a source of creosote. The nuts are known as 'mast' and are a valued feed for farm animals. Traditional use of the oil and tar for chest and skin diseases has now dwindled and this tree is currently little used in medicine. It is possible that further research may revive the former treatments or reveal new uses for this monumental tree.

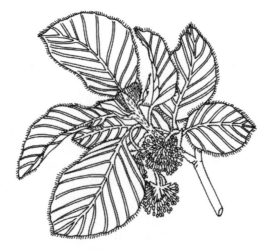

> ### Flower remedy
>
> Beech is used as one of the Bach Flower Remedies; indicated for those who 'feel the need to see more good and beauty in all that surrounds them'.

PHYTOCHEMICALS
Oil Fixed oil.
Tar Distilled beech tar yields creosote.

ACTIONS
The tar is believed to be antiseptic and expectorant.

INDICATIONS
Externally chronic bronchitis, skin diseases (including psoriasis), wet coughs.

PREPARATIONS
Internally Bach Flower Remedy.
Externally The oil and tar are not readily available.

CAUTIONS
Beech has largely fallen out of use and should only be used on expert professional advice.

Ficus carica

COMMON NAME Common fig.
PLANT FAMILY Moraceae.

RELATED SPECIES *F. benghalensis*; *F. cotinifolia*; *F. indica*; *F. insipida*; *F. lacor*; *F. religiosa*.

RANGE South-west Asia, the Mediterranean.

PARTS USED Fruit, leaves.

OVERVIEW
This small tree is well-known for its edible fruit. And for the strategic use of its leaves in the Garden of Eden! It was held sacred by the Romans and there is much mythology surrounding it . A gentle laxative preparation, 'syrup of figs', is made from it, and this is suitable even for children. A stronger preparation, 'Compound Syrup of Figs' was made containing senna and rhubarb in addition to figs. The latex (milky juice from the stem) is used for warts. The latex of a

related species (*F. insipida*) and several other types of fig are used to treat worm and other parasite infestations. The leaves have been studied in the treatment of insulin-dependent diabetes where they have shown a blood sugar lowering effect. Traditionally, the leaves of a related species, *F. benghalensis* (the banyan tree), have been used by Ayurvedic practitioners to treat diabetes.

PHYTOCHEMICALS
Enzymes, flavonoids, sugars, vitamins (A, B, C, D).

ACTIONS
Fruit Demulcent, gentle expectorant, mild laxative, nutritive.
Leaves Hypoglycaemic.

INDICATIONS
Internally Constipation, irritable coughs, in convalescence as a restorative food.

PREPARATIONS
Internally Fruit, eaten fresh or dried. To supplement conventional control of diabetes a decoction of fig leaves may be taken with breakfast.

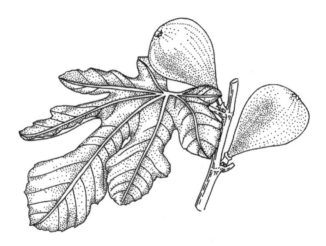

CAUTIONS
A light-sensitive skin reaction can occur if fresh fig juice is applied to the skin and the skin is then exposed to sunlight. Wash your hands after picking or eating fresh fruit. Fig leaves may be of benefit in non-insulin-dependent diabetes as a supplementary dietary control. They are not a substitute for insulin in insulin-dependent diabetes.

Ficus religiosa

COMMON NAMES Peepalbanti; peepul; sacred fig; bo-tree; bodhi.
PLANT FAMILY Moraceae.

RELATED SPECIES see *F. carica*.

RANGE Southern Asia, India.

PARTS USED Bark, fruit, leaves.

OVERVIEW
As the species name *religiosa* suggests this tree is held to be sacred in its native habitat. The Buddha is said to have achieved enlightenment while meditating under a bodhi tree. It is capable of living till a great age (up to 2,000 years). Research has supported the traditional uses of this fascinating tree for respiratory disorders such as asthma.

PHYTOCHEMICALS
Bark Tannin.
Fruit Zinc.

ACTIONS
Bark, leaves Antibacterial, astringent.
Fruit Laxative.

INDICATIONS
Internally
Fruit Asthma, constipation.
Bark, leaves Diarrhoea and dysentery, skin diseases.

PREPARATIONS
Internally The fruit is eaten. Bark and leaves are decocted.

CAUTIONS
None found.

Fraxinus excelsior

COMMON NAME Ash.
PLANT FAMILY Oleaceae.

RELATED SPECIES *F. americana* (American white ash); *F. chinensis*; *F. ornus* (manna ash).

NOT TO BE CONFUSED WITH bitter ash (*Picrasma excelsa*); mountain ash (*Sorbus aucuparia*); prickly ash (*Zanthoxylum americanum*).

RANGE Europe.

PARTS USED Leaves, bark, fruits.

OVERVIEW

This elegant tree is rarely used in medicine today but it was formerly valued for treating malaria as a substitute for Cinchona bark. In recent times it has come to attention as a constituent of an effective anti-inflammatory medicine (this includes ash bark mixed with the tree *Populus tremula* and the herb *Solidago virgaurea*). The timber is very flexible and has been used for many purposes. Green ash was traditionally used to form the curved tops of gypsy caravans. It burns well and with very little smoke, making it an excellent source of fuel. The fruits ('keys') have been pickled in vinegar and used as a food.

PHYTOCHEMICALS

Coumarins, flavonoids, tannins.

ACTIONS

Astringent, anti-inflammatory.

INDICATIONS

Internally Ash bark may be of value as part of a regime of treatment for arthritis and rheumatism.

PREPARATIONS

Internally Decoction of the bark. Tablets containing ash as part of an anti-inflammatory preparation.

CAUTIONS

None found.

Galipea officinalis

(also known as *G. cusparia*)
COMMON NAME Angostura.
PLANT FAMILY Rutaceae.

RANGE Tropical Central and South America.

PART USED Bark.

OVERVIEW

This small evergreen rainforest tree was the source of angostura bitters used to flavour soft and alcoholic drinks. The bitters were originally made in Angostura in Venezuela as a treatment for fevers. Current commercially available angostura bitters no longer contain the bark of this tree. The bark was also used as a fish poison; it is a sedative and makes them easier to catch! Medicinally it is a digestive tonic for poor digestion and spasmodic conditions of the intestines. It also continues to be used to treat fevers.

PHYTOCHEMICALS

Alkaloids (including cusparine); bitter principle; volatile oil.

ACTIONS

Antispasmodic, bitter, cholagogue, (cathartic and emetic in large doses).

INDICATIONS

Internally Decreased appetite, dysentery, fevers.

PREPARATIONS

Internally Decoction or tincture.

CAUTIONS

Can cause diarrhoea and vomiting in large doses.

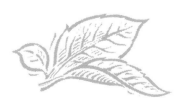

Garcinia hanburyi

COMMON NAME Gamboge.
PLANT FAMILY Guttiferae.

RELATED SPECIES There are around 200 *Garcinia* species, a number of which also have medicinal uses including: *G. bracteata*, *G. cambogia*, *G. cowa*, *G. gerrardii*, *G. kola*, *G. livingstonei*, *G. mangostana*, *G. morella*, *G. pseudoguttifera*, *G. vilersiana*, *G. xanthochymus*.

RANGE India.

PARTS USED Gum, resin.

OVERVIEW

Gamboge is the name given to the resin that can be tapped from the bark of this tree. The resin yields an orange dye used in watercolour painting and also for dyeing Buddhist robes. It is a very strong laxative used for severe constipation. Although *Garcinia hanburyi* has limited usefulness due to its potential toxicity many other species of *Garcinia* are used therapeutically. *G. cambogia* has been given to help achieve weight loss. A clinical trial did not show any effectiveness for it in promoting weight loss but this trial only gave patients the active constituent of *G. cambogia* (hydroxycitric acid), not the whole plant preparation. *G. cowa* may be of value against malaria. The leaves of *G. gerrardii* are used in Zulu medicine for earache. *G. mangostana* has shown some signs of being beneficial in treating the human immunodeficiency virus (HIV).

PHYTOCHEMICALS

Resin, gum.

ACTIONS

Purgative (strong laxative).

INDICATIONS

Internally Constipation.

PREPARATIONS

Internally Decoction or tincture of resin.

CAUTIONS

This tree is potentially toxic. The resin can cause nausea, vomiting and abdominal pain. Only to be taken on expert professional advice.

Ginkgo biloba

COMMON NAME Maidenhair tree.
PLANT FAMILY Ginkgoaceae.

RANGE Originating from China.

PARTS USED Primarily the leaves, but also seeds.

OVERVIEW

Ginkgo biloba is a remarkable tree, incredibly ancient (fossilized remains of Ginkgo have been dated as 180 million years old), it is the only species in its family (at least 6 species are extinct). It is an elegant and graceful deciduous tree that can live for over 1,000 years in the right conditions. 'Ginkgo' is Japanese for 'silver apricot', which refers to the fruit. It is widely planted along streets and in parks and is tolerant of sulphur dioxide. The male species is more commonly planted because the seeds (ginkgo nuts) of the females have an unpleasant smell. Ginkgo is best known medicinally for improving blood circulation and oxygen delivery to the brain, which can improve mental functioning including problem solving functions and memory. It also increases circulation to the limbs, easing feelings of coldness, improving the ability to walk further, and reducing painful cramps in the legs (intermittent claudication). The beneficial effects on the circulation also help prevent impaired vision in the elderly. It also helps to lower blood cholesterol, and reduce the risk of heart disease. Ginkgo can be taken safely on a long-term basis. It normally takes around 6 weeks of continued use for the benefits to manifest.

PHYTOCHEMICALS

Principally flavonoids and terpenoids. Biflavones, bilobalide, catechins, flavones, flavonol glycosides, ginkgolides, ketones, steroids.

ACTIONS

Anti-ageing, anti-allergenic, anti-asthmatic, anti-inflammatory, antioxidant, anti-PAF (platelet-activating factor), cardioprotective, circulatory stimulant (especially to the brain and limbs), lowers cholesterol.

INDICATIONS

Internally Used to treat many conditions, including:
Asthma The anti-PAF action decreases allergic reactions leading to less bron-

choconstriction and inflammation in the lungs. This eases chest tightness and wheezing. Ginkgo can be used to treat asthma in both adults and children.

Dementia Ginkgo is especially useful when introduced in the early stages of this disorder. It can be of benefit in both senile dementia and Alzheimer's disease.

Deteriorating vision This can be helped when the problem is due to a circulatory disorder affecting the retina of the eye. It may help senile macular degeneration.

Disordered limb sensations Problems with the limbs, such as feelings of coldness, cramping, numbness and tingling, may be helped by taking Ginkgo. Intermittent claudication and Raynaud's disease have also been shown to respond favourably.

Impaired mental and general cerebral functioning Ginkgo can improve alertness, communication, concentration, memory, orientation, and reduce absentmindedness, anxiety, confusion, dizziness and fatigue, particularly in older people.

Stroke recovery Ginkgo can improve recovery from strokes. It can speed the time it takes to regain normal functioning.

Tinnitus and hearing impairment Reduced hearing ability and the unpleasant noises heard in tinnitus may be helped due to improving circulation within the ear and brain.

PREPARATIONS AND DOSAGE
Internally
Standardized extract Most of the clinical trials involving Ginkgo have used specially standardized and enriched extracts containing concentrated amounts of the most active chemical constituents, the flavonoids and terpenoids. The daily dose is about 120mg of a 50:1 standardized extract (equivalent to about 30mg flavone glycoside and 10mg terpenoids per day).

Tea A decoction of the leaves. 4–8g per day. The tea is palatable but it will not be the most pleasant thing you have ever drunk!

CAUTIONS
Leaves Ginkgo leaf preparations are generally considered safe and well tolerated. They may interact with anticoagulant (such as aspirin and warfarin) and antiplatelet medicines. They should not be taken alongside these medicines unless on the advice of an expert professional.

Seeds The seeds can cause contact dermatitis (inflammation of the skin caused by touching the seeds).

Guaiacum officinale

COMMON NAMES Lignum vitae ('wood of life'), Guaiacum.
PLANT FAMILY Zygophyllaceae.

RELATED SPECIES The berries of *G. coulteri* were used medicinally by Native American tribes. *G. sanctum* is used similarly to *G. officinale*.

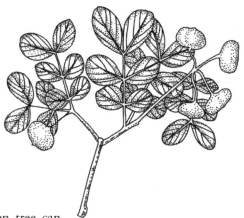

RANGE South America and West Indies. It is the national flower of Jamaica.

PARTS USED Whole heartwood cut into chips; extracted resin.

OVERVIEW

This striking blue-flowered evergreen tree can grow to 10m (30ft). It provides a very hard water-resistant timber. The whole heartwood or the isolated resin is used in medicine. The resin is obtained by heating the cut heartwood or evaporating the heartwood extract. It has been used formerly for treating wet coughs, lung congestion and influenza but is primarily used today for arthritis. It gained a reputation for treating syphilis in the sixteenth century and was in great demand for some time. Unfortunately, partly due to its fame in treating sexually transmitted disease, this tree has been over-harvested and is now threatened in the wild. For this reason its use cannot be advised unless acquired from a certified cultivated source. This is a great pity because it is one of the most useful remedies for treating osteo- and rheumatoid arthritis. Other anti-inflammatory trees, such as *Boswellia serrata*, provide a good substitute.

Conservation

G. coulteri is classed as being on the verge of becoming vulnerable to extinction. Both *G. officinale* and *G. sanctum* though are both classed as endangered species, meaning they face a very high risk of becoming extinct in the wild in the near future.

PHYTOCHEMICALS

Guaiacol, phenolic lignans, pigment, resin (18–25%), saponins, vanillin.

ACTIONS

Anti-inflammatory, diaphoretic, mild diuretic, gentle expectorant, weak laxative.

INDICATIONS

Internally Ankylosing spondylitis, arthritis (osteo-arthritis and rheumatoid arthritis), gout, rheumatism. The anti-inflammatory action of Guaiacum applies in all of these conditions. In addition, its mild detoxifying activity (removing waste products of metabolism via the bowel, kidneys and skin) helps to improve joint and muscle function. In rheumatism the diaphoretic effect probably serves to warm the circulation in the muscles helping them to relax. Guaiacum has a reputation for treating certain skin problems such as boils and psoriasis, probably due to a combination of anti-inflammatory and detoxifying actions. However, it is not suitable for treating allergic skin conditions such as atopic eczema.

Externally Guaiacum is useful in tonsillitis, where it reduces inflammation. It also probably has an antiseptic action since most highly resinous compounds stimulate the immune system when applied locally.

PREPARATIONS

Internally Use the tincture for treating arthritis, rheumatism and skin disorders. It is usually made at a strength of 1:5 90% (a high alcohol content is required to optimally extract the resinous compounds). Take 1–2ml three times a day in a glass of warm water with meals.

Externally Gargle.

CAUTIONS

Resins can be irritating to the stomach, therefore avoid Guaiacum in cases of stomach sensitivity (this side effect can normally be avoided by taking the medicine with food). Avoid the resin touching the skin, it may cause contact dermatitis.

Guarea rusbyi

COMMON NAME Cocillana.
PLANT FAMILY Meliaceae.

RELATED SPECIES These include *G. guidonia*, which is anti-inflammatory and antiviral; *G. macrophylla* which is purgative. There are around 170 *Guarea* species of trees and shrubs, 150 in tropical America and 20 in Africa.

RANGE Eastern Andes.

PART USED Bark.

OVERVIEW

Several different species of *Guarea* are used in medicine and it is often hard to tell them apart. The species *G. rusbyi* is usually given as the tree from which cocillana (the dried bark) is taken but it is likely that many different *Guarea* trees are used.

Cocillana is used to treat conditions of the chest such as bronchitis. At higher doses it can cause vomiting, it is said to act much like the herb Ipecacuanha, which is used in conventional medicine to cause vomiting in children or adults who have swallowed poisons.

PHYTOCHEMICALS
Alkaloids, anthraquinones, fixed oil, flavonols, resins, volatile oil.

ACTIONS
Emetic (at high doses), expectorant.

INDICATIONS
Internally Bronchitis, congestive coughs.

PREPARATIONS
Internally Decoction or tincture of dried bark.

CAUTIONS
Can cause vomiting. Only to be taken on expert professional advice.

Guazuma ulmifolia

COMMON NAMES Bay cedar; mutamba; pixoy; tapaculo; West Indian elm.
PLANT FAMILY Sterculiaceae.

RANGE South American tropical rainforest.

PARTS USED Bark, leaves, (root occasionally).

OVERVIEW
This is a rainforest plant that can be encountered as a shrub or medium-sized tree growing to around 12m (40ft) tall. Research showing antibacterial qualities backs up traditional use for boils and other skin infections. It has been used for many conditions throughout South America including asthma, bronchitis, during childbirth, for kidney diseases and for fevers. Traditional preparations have proven effective in controlling blood sugar levels in tests and they may be of use in controlling diabetes.

PHYTOCHEMICALS
Alkaloids, caffeine (leaf), proanthocyanidins, tannins, terpenes.

ACTIONS
Antibacterial, astringent, possibly cytotoxic.

INDICATIONS
Internally Asthma, diarrhoea, dysentery, fever, prostate problems.
Externally Skin infections.

PREPARATIONS
Internally Decoction of the bark taken by mouth.
Externally Applied to the skin as a bath in infections.

CAUTIONS
None found.

Hagenia abyssinica

COMMON NAMES Koso; kousso.
PLANT FAMILY Rosaceae.

RANGE Eastern Africa.

PART USED Flowers.

OVERVIEW
The flowers of this beautiful African tree have been used to treat infestation with worms for many centuries. Recent research suggests that there may also be antispasmodic and antitumor effects. However, like most antiparasitic plants, this tree needs to be used with great care as it can cause health problems. In Ethiopia its use has been associated with deterioration in eyesight.

PHYTOCHEMICALS
Kosins including protokosin and kosotoxin; these are phloroglucinol derivatives.

ACTIONS
Anthelmintic.

INDICATIONS
Internally Traditionally used to treat tapeworm infestation given in combination with a strong laxative.

PREPARATIONS
Internally Infusion of the flowers.

CAUTIONS
This tree is potentially toxic and should only be used on expert professional advice.

Hamamelis virginiana

COMMON NAMES Witch hazel; witchhazel.
PLANT FAMILY Hamamelidaceae.

NOT TO BE CONFUSED WITH European hazel, Corylus avellana. The leaves have some similarity but the species are unrelated.

RANGE East and North America.

PARTS USED Bark, leaves.

OVERVIEW

This elegant North American tree is widely grown as a decorative garden species. It has distinctive flowers, which are like tangled balls of yellow petals, and attractive foliage. It is famous as the source of distilled witch hazel water, which is one of the few traditional herbal preparations that has survived and is still widely available in pharmacies. Several Native American tribes used it – the Cherokee applied it to sores and grazes and the Iroquois used it to prevent bleeding following childbirth. The Mohegans used sticks as divining rods to seek out water or buried treasure. Witch hazel was formerly frequently taken by mouth to treat many internal disorders but is now mainly applied externally to various conditions appearing on the skin. A recent development has been the increased use of witch hazel in cosmetic skin creams to help prevent skin ageing and wrinkling.

Treatment tip – Piles (haemorrhiods)

Witch hazel cream is excellent for treating haemorrhoids (piles); apply to the piles at least twice a day. It can be combined with horse chestnut (*Aesculus hippocastanum*) for this purpose too.

PHYTOCHEMICALS

Flavonoids, tannins (principally hydrolysable tannins in the bark and condensed tannins in the leaves), volatile oil.

ACTIONS

Antihaemorrhagic, anti-inflammatory, astringent, vasoconstrictive.

INDICATIONS

Internally Diarrhoea. Period pain, heavy menstrual bleeding. At one time, witch hazel was used for gynaecological conditions particularly painful periods and heavy bleeding either during the period or following childbirth (post-partum haemorrhage). The tannins help to reduce blood loss.

Externally Acne, boils, bites and stings, bleeding gums and mouth ulcers, bruises, burns and scalds, conjunctivitis, eczema (the exudative or 'wet' type of eczema responds well to witch hazel. It should not be applied to 'dry' eczema – the fragile, sensitive, dry skin type of eczema), haemorrhoids, phlebitis, sore throat, tonsillitis, varicose veins, wounds.

PREPARATIONS

Internally Decoction or tincture of leaves or bark.

Externally

Cream/ointment Apply to haemorrhoids and varicose veins several times (2–6) daily.

Compress Apply the decocted leaf or bark as a compress to acne, boils, burns, scalds.

Distilled water Has a cooling and anti-inflammatory effect. Apply topically to acne, bites and stings, boils, wet eczema, haemorrhoids. Often used as a make-up remover.

Eyewash Use the carefully strained decoction or diluted tincture as an eyebath for conjunctivitis.

Gargle Gargle with the decoction or tincture for sore throats and tonsillitis.

Mouthwash Use the decoction or tincture held in the mouth for bleeding gums and ulceration.

Suppository Can be given to treat haemorrhoids and rectal bleeding. Strength should be 0.1–1g of witch hazel extract per suppository, inserted three times a day.

Wash For minor wounds use the decoction as a wash to rinse the wound to clean it and promote healing. Once the skin has begun to heal over switch to using the cream to continue the process.

CAUTIONS

The leaves and bark are mainly used externally and are generally safe and well tolerated. Internal use should be only on expert professional advice as tannins can prevent absorption of vital nutrients.

Hippophae rhamnoides

COMMON NAME Sea buckthorn; sallow thorn.
PLANT FAMILY Elaeagnaceae.

NOT TO BE CONFUSED WITH alder buckthorn (*Rhamnus frangula*); Californian buckthorn (*cascara sagrada*) (*Rhamnus purshiana*); common or purging buckthorn (*Rhamnus cathartica*). Sea buckthorn is in an entirely different family to these trees.

RANGE Europe to Northern China.

PART USED Berries.

OVERVIEW
Sea buckthorn grows principally in sandy coastal areas. Its fruits (berries) can be eaten and they have been used to flavour fish sauce. It is the berries that are used medicinally. They are vivid orange and rich in vitamin C. An oil can be extracted from the berry flesh and seeds, this has been used in the Ukraine to treat burns and leg ulcers.

PHYTOCHEMICALS
Flavonoids, vitamin C.

ACTIONS
Enhances immune resistance, vulnerary.

INDICATIONS
Internally Infections and convalescence after illness (the immune enhancing properties can be of help here).
Externally Burns and skin ulcers.

PREPARATIONS
Internally Decoction of the berries.
Externally Ointment.

CAUTIONS
None found.

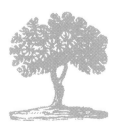

Hymenaea courbaril

COMMON NAMES Anami gum; Brazilian copal; jatoba.
PLANT FAMILY Leguminosae.

RELATED SPECIES *H. oblongifolia*; *H. parvifolia* are both used medicinally.

RANGE Tropical America (Central and South America, particularly in the Amazon).

PARTS USED Bark, leaves, resin.

OVERVIEW
This is a huge rainforest tree growing up to 30m (100ft) high. Its fruits are edible and the resinous gum obtained from it is used to make incense and varnish. It is popular as a source of medicines for many rainforest tribes, being employed in a wide number of illnesses including arthritis, asthma, coughs, cystitis, hepatitis. Traditionally, it has been seen as a tonic, helping to improve energy levels and strength, and to enhance resistance to fatigue.

PHYTOCHEMICALS
Flavonoids, phenols, terpenes.

ACTIONS
Possible adaptogen, antibacterial, antifungal, hepatoprotective.

INDICATIONS
Internally Prostatitis. Traditional indications suggest it may be useful in a large number of other infectious and inflammatory conditions.
Externally Athlete's foot.

PREPARATIONS
Internally Decoction.

CAUTIONS
None found.

Ilex aquifolium

COMMON NAMES Holly; Holy tree.
PLANT FAMILY Aquifoliaceae.

RELATED SPECIES *I. opaca* (American holly);
I. paraguaiensis (yerba mate); *I. verticillata*
(common winterberry).

RANGE Europe, Mediterranean.

PARTS USED Bark, berries, leaves, roots.

OVERVIEW

An evergreen tree with sharp thorny leaves and
bright crimson berries, holly has an unmistak-
able appearance. It has been viewed as a sacred tree
for many centuries; brought into the house
to offer protection and the promise of new life at
midwinter, it is a feature of Christmas celebrations.
The wood is white and beautiful and it burns with a bright
white flame and can be used as fuel even when freshly har-
vested. Holly is rarely used medicinally at present, but in the past the leaves were
esteemed as a remedy for infectious diseases including malaria and smallpox. In
North America the Micmac tribe used the roots for coughs and tuberculosis.

PHYTOCHEMICALS

Bitter (ilicin), caffeic acid, theobromine (leaf).

ACTIONS

Leaves Diaphoretic, diuretic.
Berries Emetic, purgative, vulnerary.

INDICATIONS

Internally Catarrh, fevers, pleurisy,
rheumatism.
Externally Wounds.

Flower remedy

Holly is one of the Bach
Flower Remedies, being
given to 'those who are
sometimes attacked by
thoughts of such kind as
jealousy, envy, revenge,
suspicion'.

PREPARATIONS

Internally Leaves as a Decoction. Bach Flower Remedy.
Externally Berries are powdered and dusted over wounds to halt bleeding.

CAUTIONS

The berries can cause vomiting, diarrhoea and drowsiness.

Ilex paraguaiensis

COMMON NAMES Yerba maté; maté; Paraguay tea; Brazilian tea.
PLANT FAMILY Aquifoliaceae.

RELATED SPECIES see *I. aquifolium*. The leaves of *I. guayusa* (guayusa, Peru), *I. verticillata* (feverbark, North America) and *I. vomitoria* (yaupon, East and North America) are also used to make teas.

RANGE Paraguay and parts of Argentina and Brazil.

PART USED Leaves.

Conservation

Although *I. paraguaiensis* is widely cultivated, it is also harvested from the wild leading to it being on the verge of becoming at risk of extinction in the wild in some areas. Try to buy maté from guaranteed cultivated sources.

OVERVIEW

Yerba maté is a large shrub or small tree; its leaves are used widely as a tea, providing the main daily beverage for many South Americans. Like China tea it contains stimulating substances such as caffeine and it is rich in tannins. It is principally seen as an item of the normal diet but is also used as a medicine for rheumatic pain and a variety of other disorders. A study showed that its antioxidant activity was stronger than that of vitamin C. The presence of caffeine means that yerba maté cannot be viewed as being a totally healthy beverage, but its caffeine content is less than that of either tea or coffee.

PHYTOCHEMICALS

Caffeine, saponins, tannins, theobromine, vitamin C, volatile oil.

ACTIONS

Antioxidant, diaphoretic, diuretic, stimulant.

INDICATIONS

Internally Depression (mild), fatigue, rheumatism.

PREPARATIONS

Internally The leaves are prepared by infusion as a tea.

CAUTIONS

Avoid in cases of stress, tension, insomnia and irritability where the stimulant effects may add to these problems.

Illicium verum

COMMON NAMES Star anise; Chinese anise.
PLANT FAMILY Illiciaceae.

RELATED SPECIES *I. anisatum* (Japanese anise).

NOT TO BE CONFUSED WITH *Pimpinella anisum* (aniseed), this herb has a volatile oil similar in composition to that of star anise.

RANGE China, Vietnam.

PARTS USED Fruits, and volatile oil distilled from them.

OVERVIEW
The star-shaped fruits of this evergreen tree are a delicious culinary spice but also an outstanding example of the beauty of plant architecture. They work primarily on the digestive system, gently warming the circulation, relaxing the muscles and improving digestive functioning. They are helpful for spasmodic, tense digestive problems such as colic and excessive wind. Chewed after meals they sweeten the breath. Star anise also is of benefit in several respiratory disorders and the oil inhalation is useful to clear congestion of the head and sinuses.

Treatment tip – Indigestion and nasal catarrh

If you are prone to bouts of indigestion or nasal catarrh you might find taking star anise tea helpful. Place 2–3 of the fruits in a cup and pour on just boiled water, leave to brew for 5 minutes with a saucer over the top to prevent the volatile oil from escaping. Take the tea hot and savour its exotic spicy aroma as you drink.

PHYTOCHEMICALS
Volatile oil (containing mainly trans-anethole; also caryophyllene and estragole).

ACTIONS
Antiseptic, aromatic digestive, carminative, expectorant.

INDICATIONS
Internally Coughs, flatulence, intestinal colic, rheumatism, upper respiratory tract infections.
Externally Abdominal pain (due to indigestion or trapped wind), catarrh, chest infections, sinusitis.

PREPARATIONS

Internally Decoction or infusion of the fruits drunk as a tea. Tincture diluted in water and sipped.

Externally The pure volatile oil can be used as an inhalation or applied externally (diluted in a carrier oil) as a chest rub or abdominal massage for digestive pain.

CAUTIONS

The volatile oil of Japanese aniseed contains the potentially toxic chemical saffrole but that of star anise does not.

Juglans cinerea

COMMON NAMES Butternut; white walnut.
PLANT FAMILY Juglandaceae.

RELATED SPECIES *J. californica* (California walnut); *J. nigra* (black walnut); *J. regia* (walnut).

RANGE East and North America.

PART USED Bark (inner part of).

OVERVIEW

The butternut is a graceful deciduous tree bearing edible seeds (nuts). It has been used as a food and medicine by several Native American tribes. The Cherokee used it to treat toothache, the Potawatomi saw it as a tonic and the Iroquois employed it widely for urinary pain, to kill worms, and to stop bleeding from

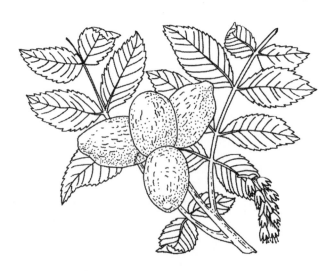

wounds. Today it is mostly valued in treating skin problems where its cleansing effects on the gallbladder, liver and digestive system help to promote good skin tone.

PHYTOCHEMICALS
Naphthoquinones (including juglone), tannins, volatile oil.

ACTIONS
Cholagogue, depurative, laxative.

INDICATIONS
Internally Constipation; skin disorders such as acne, eczema, psoriasis.

PREPARATIONS
Internally Decoction or tincture of the bark taken by mouth.

CAUTIONS
Butternut has been used traditionally to induce labour so it should only be used in pregnancy on professional advice.

Juglans regia

COMMON NAMES Walnut; English walnut.
PLANT FAMILY Juglandaceae.

RELATED SPECIES see *J. cinerea* (butternut).

RANGE South East Europe, Western Asia.

PARTS USED Bark, leaves, seeds (walnuts).

OVERVIEW
Walnut is a handsome medium to large deciduous tree. It is most well-known for its edible brain-like seeds, walnuts, surely one of the most delicious of all nuts. The wood is beautiful and was formerly highly-prized and widely used for furniture making but has largely been superseded by mahogany, which is less susceptible to woodworm. A dye is made from the husks, and oil from the seeds is used in the manufacture of paint. Unripe walnuts were once used to treat worm infestations. The leaves are presently used for skin conditions such as acne and psoriasis, and also to relieve constipation. They stimulate the liver and help to detoxify the body. The bark has been used as a toothbrush and a study has shown that it is antibacterial and may help to prevent dental caries, plaque and gum disease.

Flower remedy

Walnut is one of the Bach Flower Remedies, it is included under the category of remedies for 'oversensitivity to influences and ideas' and is said to give 'constancy and protect from outside influences'.

PHYTOCHEMICALS
Leaves Flavonoids, naphthoquinones (principally juglone), tannins, volatile oil.

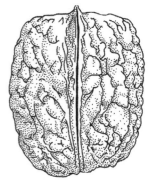

ACTIONS
Bark Antimicrobial, astringent.
Leaves Astringent, depurative, expectorant, laxative.
Seeds Nutritive.

INDICATIONS
Internally Skin disorders such as acne, eczema, psoriasis; respiratory disorders including asthma and coughs; as a general nutritive to promote health and prevent disease and as a restorative in convalescence.

PREPARATIONS
Internally
Leaves Decoction or tincture taken by mouth.
Flowers Bach Flower Remedy.
Seeds The seeds eaten fresh or dried.
Externally The decoction can also be applied externally to eczema and herpes infections.

CAUTIONS
None found.

Juniperus communis

COMMON NAMES Juniper; common juniper.
PLANT FAMILY Cupressaceae.

RELATED SPECIES There are around 50 *Juniperus* species, many of which have medicinal uses including *J. excelsa*; *J. occidentalis*; *J. oxycedrus* (the heartwood yields oil of Cade which is antiparasitic); *J. sabina* (savin). This species is toxic due to the prescence of podophyllotoxin.

RANGE Northern temperate region.

PARTS USED Principally the fruits (juniper berries) but the bark, roots and leafy twigs have also been used.

OVERVIEW

Though it is often encountered as a shrub juniper can grow to be a small tree. It is an evergreen conifer with dark purple aromatic berries that are used as a flavouring for gin and in cooking. Several ornamental varieties are grown including low-lying creeping versions. The leaves or twigs have been burnt as incense as part of purification ceremonies and to give protection from harm. In North America, the Southern Carrier tribe boiled up the branches and inhaled the aromatic steam to relieve chest pain and headaches and many tribes used juniper to prevent or treat colds. It is now used mainly for bladder infections (cystitis) and arthritis. But it has a far wider range of uses, also helping to warm and relax the digestive system and treat coughs and chest infections. The scent of the oil is delightful, pungent and penetrating. The taste of the berries is sweet, rich, deep and complex. Juniper is truly a marvel amongst medicinal trees.

PHYTOCHEMICALS

Flavonoids, resin, vitamin C, volatile oil (mostly monoterpenes).

ACTIONS

Analgesic, anti-inflammatory, antiseptic, aromatic digestive, carminative, diuretic, expectorant.

INDICATIONS

Internally Colds and infectious disease; cystitis; digestive disorders including colic, flatulence, abdominal pain; joint and muscle disorders; arthritis, gout, rheumatism; headaches; painful periods; respiratory problems including bronchitis, coughs and chest infections.

Externally Headaches, joint disorders (as above), respiratory problems (as above), sore throats.

PREPARATIONS

Internally The berries decocted and drunk as a tea or the tincture (made with 45% alcohol in order to retain a high percentage of the volatile oil) taken in water.

Externally The decoction and tincture of the berries can be used as a gargle for sore throats or as a mouthwash for oral infections. The pure volatile oil is used as an inhalation for respiratory problems, or as a massage oil for muscular conditions (diluted in a carrier oil), and applied in creams or lotions to painful joints. It can be applied over the temples to relieve headaches.

CAUTIONS

Due to the strong volatile oil content, juniper is traditionally not given in pregnancy and where there is kidney disease, either as a whole plant preparation or as the pure volatile oil. The validity of this caution has been questioned but it is wise not to use juniper in these conditions unless on expert professional advice.

Kigelia africana

(also known as Kigelia pinnata)
COMMON NAMES Sausage tree; umfongothi (Zulu).
PLANT FAMILY Bignoniaceae.

RANGE Tropical Africa and South Africa.

PARTS USED Bark, fruit.

OVERVIEW

Kigelia africana is a large dome-shaped tree with big attractive maroon flowers and huge (up to 1m/3ft long) sausage-shaped fruits. The fruits are truly remarkable in appearance; they are dried and powdered to make a medicinal preparation. This is mainly applied externally for sores and ulceration. The bark has shown useful antimicrobial effects and may be helpful in fighting a number of infections. A sausage tree cream is becoming popular in the west for the treatment of eczema.

PHYTOCHEMICALS

Bark Dihydroisocoumarin (kigelin), naphthaquinone (lapachol).
Fruit Dihydroisocoumarins.

ACTIONS

Bark Antimicrobial.

INDICATIONS

Internally Dysentery, and possibly for several infectious diseases.
Externally Applied externally to eczema, rheumatism, skin sores, ulcers.

PREPARATIONS
Internally Decoction of bark taken by mouth.
Externally The fruit is traditionally dried, powdered and applied to the affected areas. A cream and a lotion are also used.

CAUTIONS
None found.

Larix decidua

COMMON NAMES Larch (common or European larch).
PLANT FAMILY Pinaceae.

RELATED SPECIES *L. americana*; *L. laricina* (tamarack); *L. occidentalis* (western larch).

RANGE Europe.

PART USED Bark.

OVERVIEW
Larch is an outstandingly beautiful and elegant deciduous conifer. It has a rare, light and ethereal appearance in summertime. The sturdy, supple and straight trunks have been widely used for telegraph and tipi poles, and for fencing, amongst many other purposes. The distilled resin yields Venice turpentine. The bark of *Larix decidua* can help to treat chest infections, coughs and colds. Several other species are used medicinally; the leaves and bark of the North American *L. occidentalis* were boiled by the Ojibwa tribe to make a steam treatment for backache and headaches.

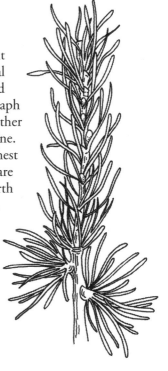

PHYTOCHEMICALS
Lignans, resin, volatile oil (including pinenes and limonene).

ACTIONS
Antiseptic, astringent, expectorant.

INDICATIONS
Internally Bronchitis, chest infections, colds, coughs, cystitis.
Externally Rheumatism, skin disorders, wounds.

PREPARATIONS
Internally Decoctions or tincture of the bark. Bach Flower Remedy derived from the flowering twigs.
Externally Decoctions of the bark applied to the affected areas as a wash or poultice. Steam baths of the leaves.

CAUTIONS
None found.

Laurus nobilis

COMMON NAMES Bay laurel; bay tree; sweet laurel; true laurel.
PLANT FAMILY Lauraceae.

NOT TO BE CONFUSED WITH Alexandrian laurel (*Calophyllum inophyllum*); cherry laurel (*Prunus laurocerasus*); Chilean laurel (*Laurelia aromatica*); Indian laurel (*Terminalia alata*); spurge laurel (*Daphne laureola*).

RANGE The Mediterranean.

PARTS USED Leaves and volatile oil distilled from the leaves.

OVERVIEW
The bay tree is an evergreen with waxy aromatic leaves that are an important culinary item. It has also long been of great symbolic importance. Leafy twigs were used to form the laurel crown worn by emperors, poets (hence the term poet laureate) and heroes. Associated with intelligence and learning, the term bachelor applied to academic degree qualifications derives from bacca-laureus, meaning 'laurel-berry'. It is a good warming antispasmodic remedy for the digestive system and is antiseptic. It is really useful to incorporate it into the diet on a regular basis by using the leaves to flavour soups, stews, sauces and gravies. The dried leaves or, even better, bruised fresh leaves can be added to olive oil and left to steep to make a very healthy salad dressing. This can also be used as a chest rub for coughs and colds and as a hair oil for dandruff.

PHYTOCHEMICALS
Volatile oil (mainly cineole, also the ester terpenyl-acetate).

ACTIONS
Antiseptic, antispasmodic, aromatic digestive, cholagogue, diaphoretic.

INDICATIONS
Internally Colic, indigestion, flatulence, lack of appetite; catarrh, coughs, colds.
Externally Bruises, chest infections, coughs, colds, dandruff, mouth ulcers, muscular stiffness, sprains.

PREPARATIONS
Internally Decoction, infusion or tincture of the leaves.
Externally Decoction as a wash for dandruff. Poultice for bruises. Volatile oil mixed with a carrier oil as a massage for chest infections, coughs, colds, muscle stiffness and sprains. It can be applied sparingly to mouth ulcers.

CAUTIONS
Avoid undiluted volatile oils coming into direct contact with the skin. Wash your hands after handling volatile oils.

Liquidambar orientalis

COMMON NAMES Levant storax; balm of Gilead.
PLANT FAMILY Hamamelidaceae.

RELATED SPECIES *L. formosana* (Chinese sweet gum); *L. styraciflua* (sweet gum); *L. taiwaniana*.

NOT TO BE CONFUSED WITH *Styrax benzoin*.

RANGE Western Asia.

PARTS USED Principally the oleo-gum resin (balsam), but also fruits, leaves, roots.

Conservation

L. orientalis var. *integriloba* and *L. orientalis* var. *orientalis* are both classed as being at risk of extinction in the wild in the medium term due to excessive harvesting for firewood and for the resin which is used in the perfume industry. If you use liquidambar, try and ensure it has come from cultivated or sustainably harvested sources.

OVERVIEW
The intriguingly named *Liquidambar* species are deciduous trees with maple or acer-like leaves that turn to spectacular shades of yellow to red in the autumn. *Liquidambar orientalis* is the source of a valuable gum known, like the tree itself, as storax. This is used as a scent as well as a medicine. The timber is valuable and the tree is widely grown particularly for the beautiful autumn leaf colours. Therapeutically it is used for coughs and colds.

PHYTOCHEMICALS
Cinnamic acid, cinnamyl cinnamate (styracin), volatile oil.

ACTIONS
Anti-inflammatory, antiseptic, expectorant.

INDICATIONS
Internally Catarrh, chest infections, colds, coughs.

PREPARATIONS
Internally Tincture diluted in water.

CAUTIONS
Resins cause burning and irritation unless properly diluted and prepared for internal use.

Liquidambar styraciflua

COMMON NAME Sweet gum.
PLANT FAMILY Hamamelidaceae.

RELATED SPECIES see *L. orientalis.*

RANGE North to Central America.

PART USED Oleo-gum resin.

OVERVIEW
Sweet gum is an attractive deciduous tree growing up to 45m (150ft) in the wild, with beautiful colourful autumn foliage. It is named after the aromatic gum resin exuded from its trunk which is used to flavour foods and tobacco and as a scent in the perfumery industry. Its timber is known as satin walnut. It is antiseptic and stimulates lung activity. It is useful for colds and chest infections.

PHYTOCHEMICALS
Resin, volatile oil.

ACTIONS
Antimicrobial, anti-inflammatory, expectorant.

INDICATIONS
Internally Asthma, colds, coughs, cystitis.
Externally Fungal infections, scabies, sore throats.

PREPARATIONS
Internally Tincture diluted in water.
Externally Cream or lotion.

CAUTIONS
Resins cause burning and irritation unless properly diluted and prepared for internal or external use.

Maclura tinctoria

COMMON NAME Toothache tree.
PLANT FAMILY Moraceae.

RELATED SPECIES *M. pomifera* (Osage orange).

NOT TO BE CONFUSED WITH *Zanthoxylum* species are also commonly known as toothache trees.

RANGE South America.

PART USED Latex.

OVERVIEW
Toothache tree is a tall rainforest canopy tree whose latex is applied to painful teeth. It appears to relieve the pain and loosen the tooth ready for extraction. Its antiseptic activity is also likely to play a role in treating any underlying infection giving rise to the toothache. Parts of the tree are also used to treat sexually transmitted diseases.

PHYTOCHEMICALS
Flavonoids.

ACTIONS
Anodyne, antiseptic, diuretic.

INDICATIONS
Internally Coughs, rheumatism, sexually transmitted disease, toothache.

PREPARATIONS
Internally For toothache the latex is applied directly to the affected tooth.

CAUTIONS
May cause loosening of healthy as well as diseased teeth.

Magnolia officinalis

COMMON NAME Magnolia tree.
PLANT FAMILY Magnoliaceae.

RELATED SPECIES *M. acuminata* (cucumber tree); *M. liliflora* (lily-flowered magnolia); *M. macrophylla* (bigleaf magnolia).

RANGE Western China.

PART USED Bark.

OVERVIEW

Magnolia trees are named after Pierre Magnol, a professor of botany and medicine who died in 1715. They have large and beautiful flowers for which they are widely cultivated as ornamental specimens. *Magnolia officinalis* is a deciduous tree whose bark (*hou po*) and flowers (*hou po hua*) have been used in Chinese medicine for thousands of years. The bark and flowers are both used to treat digestive problems though the flowers are considered weaker than the bark. Magnolol, one of the main active constituents in magnolia, has been shown to increase release of corticosteroids, which may explain the usefulness of this tree in asthma. *M. officinalis* is an ingredient in an ancient Chinese formula for treating depression called Banxia Houpo Decoction. The flower buds of a Chinese relative, *M. liliflora*, are used for nasal or sinus congestion and for headaches related to such congestion. The North American cucumber tree, *M. acuminata*, so-called because of the shape and colour of its young fruits, was used by the Cherokee tribe for digestive problems such as stomachache and diarrhoea as well as for sinus problems and toothache. It was also used for rheumatism and malaria. *M. officinalis* is classed as being on the verge of becoming vulnerable to extinction in the wild due to excessive harvesting of the bark for medicinal use. Try to buy certified cultivated or sustainably wild harvested magnolia. Several other species of magnolia used as substitutes for *M. officinalis*, such as *M. sinensis* and *M. wilsonii* are also at risk of extinction in the wild.

Treatment tip – Overindulgence

Magnolia officinalis bark tea can be drunk to relieve abdominal fullness and chest congestion associated with overindulgence in eating and drinking. It can be useful after that blow-out at the Christmas party!

PHYTOCHEMICALS
Magnolol.

ACTIONS
Bitter, aromatic digestive.

INDICATIONS
Internally Abdominal bloating and fullness, asthma, belching, diarrhoea, loss of appetite, stomachaches, vomiting.

PREPARATIONS
Internally Decoction or tincture of the bark or flowers.

CAUTIONS
The traditional view is that this herb should be used with caution in pregnancy.

Malpighia glabra

COMMON NAMES Acerola cherry; Barbados cherry.
PLANT FAMILY Malphigiaceae.

RANGE Tropical America.

PARTS USED Bark, fruit, leaves.

Treatment tip

Acerola cherry supplements provide an ideal daily nutritive support and can be taken as a general health promoter, as a preventive medicine and as a supportive measure during infections.

OVERVIEW
Acerola is a small tree with red, cherry-like, edible fruits, which are used in cooking to make jams and syrups. Unlike cherries, however, they contain several separate seeds rather than a typical cherry stone. They are one of the richest sources of vitamin C and products made from them are increasingly popular as nutritional supplements. It has long been regarded as having the highest vitamin C content of all plants although this distinction goes to the fruits of the camu camu tree (*Myricaria dubia*). Skin creams containing acerola extracts utilize its vitamin and mineral content to promote healthy looking skin tone. It was traditionally used for fevers where the immune boosting potential of vitamin C can be of great benefit.

PHYTOCHEMICALS
Nutrients Calcium, iron, niacin, pantothenic acid, protein, riboflavin, thiamine, vitamins A and C.

ACTIONS
Bark, leaves Antifungal.
Fruit Antifungal, antioxidant, nutritive, tonic.

INDICATIONS
Internally To promote good health and prevent disease; colds, influenza, fevers; as a restorative during convalescence; traditionally used for dysentery.

PREPARATIONS
Internally The fresh fruits are edible, dried fruits are decocted. A tincture can be used. A fresh juice product is available, as are several acerola supplements in capsule, tablet or powder form.

CAUTIONS
None found.

Malus species

COMMON NAMES Apple; crab apple.
PLANT FAMILY Rosaceae.

SPECIES USED The common edible apple is called *Malus domestica*, although its botanical origins are complex. There are very many varieties of this particular species known, giving a massive range of apple flavours, scents and colours. The true crab apple is *M. sylvestris*.

NOT TO BE CONFUSED WITH Apple trees were formerly classified in the *Pyrus* (pear tree) genus but are now seen as a distinct group.

RANGE Northern temperate region.

PARTS USED Bark, fruit.

OVERVIEW
This deciduous fruit tree has much history and mythology attached to it. The magical Isle of Avalon was known as the isle of apples. Mistletoe favours apple trees as a host, further enhancing their mystical reputation. Several alcoholic drinks are made from it, including cider and calvados (apple brandy). Apples come in three main types: the tart, crab apples, ordinary eating apples and cooking apples. Apples have long been associated with health (an apple a day keeps the doctor away) and chewing a raw apple provides good exercise for the teeth and gums, and the fruit acids clean the teeth. The regular drinking of cider in Normandy was associated with a low level of kidney stones in the local population. The main benefits of eating apples lies in the stimulating effect on digestion of the fruit acids, their helpfulness in causing normal bowel movements, and

their soluble fibre content which can help lower cholesterol levels thereby protecting the heart and circulation and promoting longevity.

Flower remedy

A Bach Flower Remedy is made by boiling the flowering twigs from the crab apple tree. It is indicated for 'those who feel as if they had something not quite clean about themselves'. This links with the traditional view of apples as having a cleansing effect on the body, purifying and detoxifying.

PHYTOCHEMICALS
Iron, malic acid, soluble fibre (pectin).

ACTIONS
Aperient, digestive stimulant, hypocholesterolaemic, laxative (stewed apples), nutritive.

INDICATIONS
Internally Promotion of health and prevention of disease; restorative in convalescence; healthy bowel function; constipation in people of all ages, particularly children.

PREPARATIONS
Internally Fresh apples eaten, raw or cooked, as part of a healthy diet. Dried apple rings are a good sweet food substitute, especially for children, and have a slightly laxative effect. Stewed apples make a good convalescent food.

CAUTIONS
Excessive fruit consumption can cause griping abdominal pains and diarrhoea. Crab apples cause these symptoms with ease and should not be eaten raw.

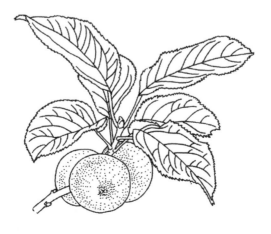

Mangifera indica

COMMON NAME Mango.
PLANT FAMILY Anacardiaceae.

RANGE India.

PARTS USED Flowers, fruits, leaves.

OVERVIEW

This large (up to 40m/130ft tall) evergreen tree is well-known for its fruit – the mango. Mangoes vary in shape and colour; they can be green, red, purple, pink and yellow. The flowers are used for chest disorders including asthma. The leaves are taken as a contraceptive but need to be used with care as they can also cause abortions. They have also shown antioxidant and antiviral activity. Above all the delicious fruits should be enjoyed as part of a healthy diet to promote general good health.

PHYTOCHEMICALS
Mangiferin, nutrients.

ACTIONS
Antimicrobial; antioxidant; possible contraceptive; emmenagogue; expectorant; nutritive.

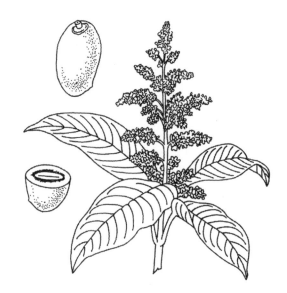

INDICATIONS
Internally
Flowers Asthma, coughs and chest infections.
Fruits Restorative following illness.

PREPARATIONS
Internally The fruit eaten raw as a part of the normal diet; leaves and flowers by decoction or infusion.

CAUTIONS
The leaves have been observed to cause abortions so should not be taken during pregnancy.

Maytenus species

COMMON NAME See under Species Used
PLANT FAMILY Celastraceae

SPECIES USED There are over 200 *Maytenus* species many of which are used as medicines, including *M. boaria; M. illicifolia* (espinheira santa); *M. laevis* (chuchuhuasca); *M. senegalensis* (red spike-thorn); *M. umbellata*.

(***Note:*** many South American species are commonly called chuchuhuasca.)

RANGE Africa and South America.

PART USED Depends on the species but mostly the bark.

OVERVIEW
Maytenus are evergreen trees and shrubs occurring in South America and Africa. There are many species and they would require a whole book to themselves to catalogue their activities and uses! A chemical called maytansine has been found in *Maytenus* species that is active against leukaemia; other potential antitumour chemicals have been identified. They offer possible starting points for new anti-cancer drugs. The roots of *M. senegalensis* are used by native tribes for pain in various parts of the body (including back, chest, and head), coughing of blood, constipation and infertility; the leaves or roots are taken for epilepsy, pneumonia and tuberculosis, snakebite and sexually transmitted disease; and the leaves are prepared to treat earache and heavy menstrual bleeding. These trees have a lot to offer us, but they need to be investigated further, especially because they contain strong plant compounds.

PHYTOCHEMICALS
Many species contain alkaloids, catechin, procyanidins, tannins, triterpenoids.

ACTIONS
M. boaria – febrifuge.
M. illicifolia – contraceptive.
M. laevis – anodyne, immunostimulant.
M. senegalensis – cytotoxic (anti-tumour).

INDICATIONS
Maytenus trees can be employed for a variety of conditions ranging from arthritic and rheumatic pain, the treatment of infections and fevers, relieving stomach complaints, and as a form of family planning through to a potential use in treating cancers.

PREPARATIONS
Most commonly, bark decoctions are utilized.

CAUTIONS
Maytenus trees contain alkaloids, so preparations should only be taken following expert professional advice.

Melaleuca alternifolia

COMMON NAME Tea tree.
PLANT FAMILY Myrtaceae.

RELATED SPECIES *M. cajuputi* (cajuput); *M. quinquenervia* (niaouli).

RANGE Australia.

PART USED Volatile oil distilled from the leaves.

OVERVIEW
Tea tree is a small to medium-sized Australian tree noted for its volatile oil (tea tree oil) which is very popular and widely used at present. Its main attributes are that it is antibacterial and antifungal. Many health and hygiene products containing tea tree oil are available including – shampoos, soaps, deodorants, lip balms and toothpastes. Tea tree can be used for many common problems, such as in a cream for athlete's foot, as a lotion for pustular spots, and diluted in vegetable oil for ringworm and other fungal skin infections. For coughs and colds it can be used as an inhalation as long as the nose and airways are not too sore, or applied diluted in a carrier oil as a rub to the chest and feet. It is of great value for treating infestation with head lice; tea tree shampoos can kill the eggs (nits) and work well combined with regular wet combing to prevent the build-up of eggs. It is a truly marvellous and versatile medicine that should find a place in everyone's first aid box.

PHYTOCHEMICALS
Volatile oil Mono and sesquiterpenes; monoterpenols (especially terpenen-4-ol); oxides (cineole).

ACTIONS
Antibacterial, antifungal, expectorant, immunostimulant.

INDICATIONS
Externally Abscesses, acne, boils, impetigo, head lice, oral and vaginal thrush, vaginitis (infection with *Trichomonas vaginalis*), respiratory infections, ringworm, sinusitis, athlete's foot.

PREPARATIONS

Externally The volatile oil is used as an inhalation, in a massage oil, as a mouth-wash (combined with an emulsifier) for oral thrush, pessary (for vaginal thrush), in shampoo (for head lice) and in lotions and creams for skin infections.

CAUTIONS

Tea tree oil should only be used internally or neat externally on expert professional advice. Do not use as an inhalation if the lining of the nose or throat is very inflamed and sore. Avoid undiluted volatile oils coming into direct contact with the skin. Allergic dermatitis (skin inflammation) reactions to tea tree oil occur quite commonly. Tea tree oil can be irritating and very drying to the skin and should only be applied in a suitable carrier oil, cream or other medium. Wash your hands after handling volatile oils.

Melaleuca cajuputi

(also known as *M. leucadendron*)
COMMON NAMES Cajuput; cajeput; swamp tea tree; white tea tree;
weeping paperbark; weeping tea tree.
PLANT FAMILY Myrtaceae.

RELATED SPECIES *M. alternifolia* (tea tree); *M. quinquenervia* (naiouli).

RANGE Northern Australia, Moluccas.

PARTS USED Volatile oil distilled from the leaves and twigs.

OVERVIEW

Cajuput comes from the Malaysian words kayu-puti, meaning 'white wood'. It has many of the same uses as tea tree oil but is more widely used as a circulatory stimulant and pain reliever, it makes a good massage oil (mixed with a carrier oil such as almond oil) for arthritic joints and stiff or rheumatic muscles.

PHYTOCHEMICALS

Oxides (mainly cineole) and monoterpenes.

ACTIONS

Analgesic, anthelmintic, antiseptic, antispasmodic, circulatory stimulant, diaphoretic, expectorant.

INDICATIONS

Internally Roundworm infestation
Externally Acne, bronchitis, colds, earache, rheumatism, skin infections, sinusitis, toothache.

PREPARATIONS
Internally Mixed with fixed oil in a capsule.
Externally The oil can be given as an inhalation, massage oil (diluted in a carrier), lotion or cream.

CAUTIONS
Cajuput oil has been used internally for parasite infestations but it should only be used internally on expert professional advice.

Melaleuca quinquenervia

(also known as *M. viridiflora*)
COMMON NAMES Niaouli.
PLANT FAMILY Myrtaceae.

RELATED SPECIES *M. alternifolia* (tea tree); *M. cajuputi* (cajuput).

RANGE Eastern Australia, New Guinea.

PART USED Volatile oil distilled from the leaves.

OVERVIEW
Niaouli is an Australian tree used, like its close relatives, for its volatile oil content. It is antiseptic like tea tree, but has a specific antiviral action, which makes it valuable for treating viral respiratory infections and colds, genital herpes and cold sores. It is very helpful for sinusitis as a steam inhalation and massaged over the sinus areas (to either side of the nose and above the eyes – being careful to avoid touching the eyes) as a lotion or cream.

PHYTOCHEMICALS
Alcohols (terpineol, viridiflorol); oxides (cineole).

ACTIONS
Anticatarrhal, anti-inflammatory, antimicrobial, antiviral, immunostimulant.

INDICATIONS
Externally Bronchitis, sinusitis, viral infections especially colds and herpes infections.

PREPARATIONS
Externally The volatile oil can be applied as an inhalation, lotion, cream or massage oil (diluted in a carrier oil).

Cautions
Avoid undiluted volatile oils coming into direct contact with the skin. Wash your hands after handling volatile oils.

Melia azedarach

Common names Ceylon mahogany; China berry; Persian lilac.
Plant family Meliaceae.

Related species *Azadirachta indica* (neem tree) is a related species, formerly described as *Melia azadirachta*. *Melia toosendan* (Sichuan pagoda tree) is used in traditional Chinese medicine for parasite infestation and as a painkiller.

Range Asia to Australia.

Parts used Bark, flowers, heartwood, leaves, roots.

Overview
This is a small deciduous tree that has a primary use as an insecticide. It has pretty scented lilac flowers and is often grown as a shade tree along streets in warm climates. Medically it is used to treat infestations with parasites, for fevers and to cause vomiting (for instance, to try and clear poisons from the body). There are several other interesting traditional uses for this tree including its possible value in cases of asthma. Research has revealed an antiviral effect from the fruits against herpes simplex virus-1, the virus that causes cold sores.

Phytochemicals
Steroids, triterpenoids.

Actions
Anthelmintic (bark, leaves); anti-inflammatory (leaves); emetic (bark, leaves, roots); emmenagogue (bark); insecticidal (leaves).

Indications
Internally
Heartwood Asthma.
Leaf Colds, constipation.
Flowers Influenza, fevers.
Roots Malaria, poisonings, worm infestation.
Externally
Leaf Eczema.
Flowers Lice infestation.

PREPARATIONS

Internally Infusions of the leaves. Bark, heartwood and roots are decocted.
Externally Infusion of leaves for eczema. Poultices of the infused flowers are applied to lice and other skin infections.

CAUTIONS

Melia preparations may cause nausea, vomiting and diarrhoea. They should not be used during pregnancy because they may cause abortions. All parts of this tree should only be taken on expert professional advice.

Morus species

PLANT FAMILY Moraceae.

SPECIES USED *Morus alba* (white mulberry); *Morus nigra* (black mulberry, common mulberry); *M. rubra* (red mulberry).

RANGE China (*Morus alba*), Western Asia (*Morus nigra*).

PARTS USED Bark, fruits, leaves, twigs.

OVERVIEW

Both the black and the white mulberry are deciduous trees with edible fruits. They are attractive trees which tend to have short thick trunks. In former times they were revered as symbolizing the quality of wisdom. The fruit of the black mulberry particularly is wonderfully juicy and delicious. Both trees have similar medicinal uses but the white mulberry, *Morus alba* has been used in Chinese medicine for a longer period of time and is better known and more widely used. This species is also grown to provide food for silkworms (they eat the leaves). The properties of the tree differ depending on which part is used; they cover a wide variety of problems. The best way to enjoy the benefits of mulberries is to eat the berries either fresh or preserved in jams and sauces. The fruits help to prevent disease by stimulating the immune system.

PHYTOCHEMICALS

M. nigra – fruit acids, pectin, vitamin C, in the fruit.
M. alba – anthocyanins, flavonoids in the leaves.

ACTIONS

Fruits In Chinese energetic terms they tonify the blood and enrich the yin; antioxidant, nutrient.
Leaves In energetic terms they expel wind, clear heat from the lungs, clear the liver and eyes, cool the blood; antioxidant.
Twigs In energetic terms they dispel wind; immunostimulant.

INDICATIONS
Internally As a restorative during recovery from illness, colds and influenza, coughs and asthma, dizziness, tinnitus (fruits); high blood pressure, joint pains, oedema (twigs).

PREPARATIONS
Internally Black mulberries eaten as part of a healthy diet. Other parts by decoction.

CAUTIONS
None found.

Myrciaria dubia

COMMON NAME Camu camu.
PLANT FAMILY Myrtaceae.

RELATED SPECIES *M. cauliflora* (jaboticaba) has edible fruits.

RANGE Amazon Basin.

PART USED Fruits.

OVERVIEW
The green and red camu camu fruits, looking like small round apples, are remarkable for their vitamin C content. They are the richest source of vitamin C yet discovered, being 30 times stronger than citrus fruits. This makes them of immense value in improving general health and supporting immune functions.

PHYTOCHEMICALS
Vitamin C.

ACTIONS
Antioxidant, immunostimulant, nutritive.

INDICATIONS
Internally Restorative remedy in convalescence; supportive treatment in colds and other infections; as a dietary supplement to prevent heart disease and other serious conditions.

PREPARATIONS
Internally The fresh fruit eaten or its juice drunk. Tablet supplements are likely to become available.

CAUTIONS
None found.

Myristica fragrans

COMMON NAME Nutmeg.
PLANT FAMILY Myristicaceae.

RANGE The Moluccas.

PARTS USED Aril (mace), seed (nutmeg), volatile oil distilled from seed.

OVERVIEW

The nutmeg tree only grows naturally in a small group of South Sea Islands called the Moluccas and known as the Spice Islands. The seed of the nutmeg tree is called nutmeg but the red covering (the aril) is known as mace. Nutmeg and mace are both used as flavourings for foodstuffs. The taste and aroma is complex and fascinating. Nowadays the medical interest in nutmeg has waned but it continues to play a role, particularly in treating digestive disorders. It warms and settles the digestive functioning. This spice is particularly useful if you suffer from a cold or sluggish stomach and bowels. It is also thought to be an aphrodisiac. Use grated nutmeg in cooking and add it to spicy hot winter drinks to improve the circulation and ward off infection.

PHYTOCHEMICALS

Fixed oils; protein; volatile oil – including monoterpenes, alcohols (including terpinen-4-ol), phenolic ethers (including safrole and myristicin).

ACTIONS

Analgesic, anti-emetic, aromatic digestive, carminative, circulatory stimulant, antispasmodic.

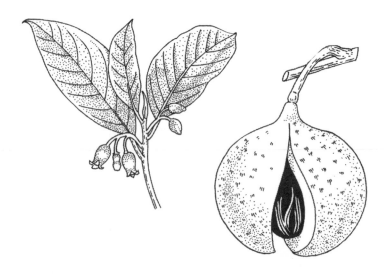

INDICATIONS
Internally Diarrhoea and dysentery, flatulence, indigestion, intestinal colic, nausea and vomiting, premature ejaculation, rheumatic and muscular pain, toothache.

PREPARATIONS
Internally Decoctions or tinctures of nutmeg are used and taken by mouth. Alternatively the grated nutmeg can be infused.
Externally A tincture applied directly to the affected tooth can help relieve toothache. The essential oil is used externally as a massage oil (diluted in a carrier oil) for rheumatic pains.

CAUTIONS
The stimulant effect of taking nutmeg can sometimes be pronounced, similar to amphetamine. Excessive use of nutmeg causes dizziness, headaches and nausea. Myristicin in the volatile oil is hallucinogenic and potentially toxic; overdose can cause convulsions, coma and death. Do not use the volatile oil internally.

Myroxylon balsamum

COMMON NAME Balsam of Tolu.
PLANT FAMILY Leguminosae.

RELATED SPECIES *Myroxylon balsamum* var. *pereirae* (Balsam of Peru).

RANGE Venezuela to Peru.

PARTS USED Oleo-resin extracted from the bark and sap wood of the trunk.

OVERVIEW
Balsam of Tolu and Balsam of Peru are two closely related large evergreen trees. Both exude a resinous compound that smells like vanilla (they are used in the perfume industry). This substance is antiseptic, and stimulates removal of mucus from the lungs. Balsam of Tolu is an ingredient in Friar's balsam and both trees are used as part of several cough syrups and mixtures. Balsam of Peru has been applied externally to treat scabies and other skin disorders. The resin can be cut up and incorporated into incense mixtures where it provides a sweet, dreamy and purifying aroma.

PHYTOCHEMICALS
Cinnamic and benzoic acids and their esters, triterpenoids, vanillin.

ACTIONS
Antiseptic, expectorant.

INDICATIONS
Internally Catarrhal and congestive conditions of the nose and lungs, coughs.

PREPARATIONS
Internally Tinctures or syrups are the best type of preparations. The tincture needs to be well diluted before drinking.

CAUTIONS
Like all resinous compounds, these balsams can be irritating to the lining of the mouth and to the digestive system, they need to be properly diluted before being taken by mouth.

Olea europea

COMMON NAME Olive.
PLANT FAMILY Oleaceae.

RELATED SPECIES *O. europea* subsp. *africana. Olea europea* is thought to be derived from this tree.

RANGE The Mediterranean.

PARTS USED Fruits (and the fixed oil expressed from them), leaves.

OVERVIEW
The olive tree is a slow-growing evergreen plant with distinctive sea grey leaves. The fruits (olives) are a well-known culinary delicacy; they can be black or green. The oil pressed from them is high in monounsaturated fatty acids and forms an important part of a diet designed to lower the risk of heart disease (the 'Mediterranean diet'). A study of 23 people with high blood pressure has shown that supplementing the diet with olive oil can lower blood pressure and reduce the need for the drugs that control high blood pressure. Cold pressed extra virgin oil is the best quality. The leaves themselves can be used to lower high blood pressure. In Africa, the Zulus use *Olea euopea* subsp. *africana* to treat urinary infections and headaches. The olive is a sacred and symbolic tree, to 'extend the olive branch' is to promote peace.

PHYTOCHEMICALS
Leaves Oleanolic acid, oleasterol, oleuropein, triterpenoid alcohols.
Oil Glycerides of linoleic and oleic acids, polyphenols.

ACTIONS
Leaves Diuretic, hypotensive.
Oil Cardioprotective, emollient, laxative (mild), nutritive.

INDICATIONS
Internally
Leaves High blood pressure.
Oil High cholesterol levels.
Externally
Oil Dandruff, for dry and poorly nourished skin, to soften earwax.

PREPARATIONS
Internally
Fruits Eaten. Those preserved in oil are preferable to those in brine as they have a lower salt content.
Leaves Decoction or tincture.
Oil Taken unheated as a salad dressing. Makes a good replacement for butter or margarine when spread on bread.
Externally
Oil Provides a good base oil for making plant oils such as St John's wort oil. It is a good massage carrier oil, being nourishing to the skin. Massage into the scalp to treat dandruff. A couple of drops warmed in a saucer over a cup of hot water can be dropped in the ear to soften earwax.
Flowers A Bach Flower Remedy is made from the flowering twigs.

CAUTIONS
Leaf tinctures and decoctions can cause stomach irritation so should be taken just after eating meals.

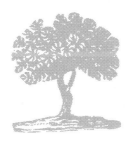

Pausinystalia johimbe

COMMON NAMES Yohimbe; johimbe.
PLANT FAMILY Rubiaceae.

RELATED SPECIES *P. macroceras*; *P. pachyceras*; *P. tillesii*.

NOT TO BE CONFUSED WITH *Puasinystalia* species are also known as *Corynanthe* species.

RANGE West Africa.

PART USED Bark.

OVERVIEW
Yohimbe is a large evergreen tree well-known as an aphrodisiac. It stimulates the heart and circulation and enhances the male erection by improving blood supply to the penis as well as improving libido. Unfortunately it has some severe drawbacks – it can exacerbate several medical conditions (particularly heart conditions) and cause unpleasant side effects such as anxiety and headaches. Fortunately there is a safer alternative to yohimbe for treating sexual disorders. This is a South American tree called muira puama (see *Ptychopetalum olacoides*).

PHYTOCHEMICALS
Alkaloids (principally yohimbine).

ACTIONS
Anaesthetic, aphrodisiac, cardiac stimulant, bitter, hypertensive.

INDICATIONS
Internally Traditionally given for poor libido and lack of sexual performance in men.

PREPARATIONS
Internally Decoctions of the bark or tablets of powdered bark. Quality control is important since analysis of yohimbe products for sale in Western health food shops has shown that many contained no yohimbine but had caffeine instead. There are legal restrictions on the availability of yohimbe in some countries.

CAUTIONS
Not to be used unless on expert professional advice. Should not be used by anyone with a heart, kidney, liver or psychiatric problem. Never to be taken by people with high blood pressure, even when this is controlled by medication. Overdose may cause psychiatric, cardiovascular and respiratory disorders.

Persea americana

COMMON NAMES avocado pear.
PLANT FAMILY Lauraceae.

RANGE Central America.

PARTS USED Fruit, leaves, seeds.

OVERVIEW

The delicious fruit of this medium to large tree is the avocado, which has been cultivated for over 10,000 years. It is as nutritious as it is tasty, containing important oils and vitamins. It is a good food source of vitamin E, which is an important anti-oxidant. Parts of the tree have been used for several medicinal purposes including for treating anaemia, liver problems, high blood pressure, colds, headaches and diabetes. It has also traditionally been used as an aphrodisiac (the fruit) and as a contraceptive (the seeds).

Treatment tip

Incorporating avocados into your diet on a regular basis will help promote healthy skin and hair and, due to its antioxidant qualities, play a role in helping to prevent cancer and heart disease. Try having avocados in salads, sandwiches, and blended into dips such as guacamole – my own recipe is to blend together avocado and tofu, adding some lemon juice, olive oil, garlic and cayenne pepper.

PHYTOCHEMICALS
Fruit Essential fatty acids, vitamin E.

ACTIONS
Fruit Antioxidant, nutritive; restorative to skin, hair and nails.
Leaves Possible hypotensive.
Seeds Possible contraceptive.

INDICATIONS
Internally
Fruit Taken in convalescence as a restorative food. Poor skin and hair texture.
Leaves Colds, fevers, high blood pressure, liver disease, painful periods.
Seeds Asthma, fertility control, snakebites.
Externally
Fruit Poor skin and hair texture.
Leaves Headaches, rheumatism, sprains.

PREPARATIONS
Internally
Fruit Eaten raw.
Leaves Decoction.
Seeds Decoction.
Externally
Fruit Mashed and applied directly to hair and skin.
Leaves A poultice is used for headaches.
Oil An oil is pressed from the avocado and provides an excellent healing carrier oil for use in massage.

CAUTIONS
Repeated use of the seeds as a contraceptive is thought to cause sterility.

Peumus boldo

COMMON NAME Boldo.
PLANT FAMILY Monimiaceae.

RANGE Chile and Peru.

PART USED Leaves.

OVERVIEW
Boldo is a small evergreen tree. Boldo leaves have been traditionally utilized to treat gallbladder and liver conditions and research now backs this up. They stimulate the gallbladder and protect the liver from toxins. Boldo offers a promising treatment for hepatitis particularly.

PHYTOCHEMICALS
Alkaloids (including boldine), flavanoids, volatile oil.

ACTIONS
Anthelmintic, antioxidant, cholagogue, choleretic, diuretic, hepatoprotective.

INDICATIONS
Internally Cystitis, gallstones and gallbladder inflammation (cholecystitis), hepatitis, worm infestation.

PREPARATIONS
Internally The leaves are decocted or a tincture can be used.

CAUTIONS

Boldo contains strong chemicals (alkaloids; ascaridole in the volatile oil) and should only be used for short periods of time (2–6 weeks). It should not be used in pregnancy. A pure boldo volatile oil can be obtained but this should be avoided as it can cause damage to the nervous system.

Phellodendron amurense

COMMON NAMES Huang bai; Amur cork-tree.
PLANT FAMILY Rutaceae.

RANGE China, Japan, Korea.

PART USED Bark.

> ## Conservation
>
> *Phellodendron amurense* var. *wilsonii* is causing concern since forest clearances and overxploitation for medicinal use have significantly reduced its numbers in the wild.

OVERVIEW

Amur cork-tree is a deciduous Asian tree with elegant leaves used in traditional Chinese medicine. *Phellodendron* refers to the corky bark of this tree (*phellos* = cork, *dendron* = tree). The bark is the part used and the inner layer of it is coloured yellow. The bark is considered to be bitter and cold and is given to treat damp-heat disorders such as diarrhoea and vaginal discharge. It also drains kidney fire making it useful in conditions involving sweating. It has an antimicrobial effect due to the presence of berberine.

PHYTOCHEMICALS

Alkaloids, including berberine, magnoflorine, phellodendrine.

ACTIONS

Antimicrobial, bitter.

INDICATIONS

Internally Diarrhoea, dysentery, night sweats.
Externally Vaginal and cervical infections with Trichomonas vaginalis.

PREPARATIONS
Internally The bark is decocted and taken by mouth.
Externally The decoction given as a vaginal douche for *Trichomonas* infection.

CAUTIONS
May rarely cause a skin rash.

Picrasma excelsa

COMMON NAMES Quassia; Jamaica quassia; bitter ash; bitter wood.
PLANT FAMILY Simaroubaceae.

NOT TO BE CONFUSED WITH Several related species of *Picrasma* cause confusion by having the word quassia connected with them, including *Quassia amara*, *Quassia cedron* and *Quassia indica*. These are all in the same family but are different species. *Picrasma ailanthoides* is Japanese quassia.

RANGE West Indies

PART USED Wood.

Conservation

P. excelsa is now classed as a vulnerable species meaning that it is at high risk of becoming extinct in the wild in the medium term. Try and buy quassia that is certified as cultivated or sustainably harvested.

OVERVIEW
Quassia is a handsome ash-like tree growing to 25m (80ft) in height. The wood of the trunk is dried and cut up for use as a medicine (quassia chips). It tastes intensely bitter and has been used as a tonic for the digestive system to stimulate appetite and help recovery from illness. It has also been used as an insecticide and to flavour alcoholic and soft drinks. Quassia is a traditional remedy for malaria. It is also very useful for treating infestation with head lice. A teaspoon of the tincture can be mixed with a regular amount of shampoo or conditioner and applied to the hair; leave on for 5 minutes before rinsing. Repeat this each day for two weeks. Alternatively, you can make a decoction of the wood and use this as a rinse after every hair wash. The hair should be wet combed every day as well to remove the lice.

PHYTOCHEMICALS
Alkaloids, quassinoids.

ACTIONS
Anthelmintic, antipyretic, bitter, tonic.

INDICATIONS
Internally Lack of appetite, constipation, to aid convalescence, dyspepsia, fevers, worm infestation.
Externally Head lice infestation

PREPARATIONS
Internally Decoction or tincture of the wood
Externally Decoction used as a wash for head lice or given as an enema for threadworm infestation. The tincture can be combined with shampoo and used for treating head lice.

CAUTIONS
Excessive consumption of quassia can cause stomach irritation, nausea and vomiting.

Pimenta dioica

COMMON NAMES Allspice, pimento, Jamaica pepper.
PLANT FAMILY Myrtaceae.

RELATED SPECIES *Pimenta racemosa* (bay rum tree).

RANGE Central America, West Indies.

PART USED Fruit.

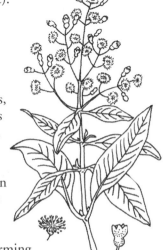

OVERVIEW
Pimenta dioica is an evergreen tree with brown fruits, known as allspice because their flavour contains hints of several spice tastes including cinnamon, cloves, juniper and nutmeg. They are harvested just after they reach full size while still unripe as they lose their complexity of aroma and taste when ripe. Allspice has been used to flavour alcoholic drinks such as Benedictine, Chartreuse and mulled wine. Although mainly used in the kitchen, allspice has medicinal effects on the digestive system, warming

and relaxing it, improving absorption of nutrients and reducing flatulence. If you don't already use allspice, try incorporating it into your cooking and add a pinch to spicy hot winter drinks.

PHYTOCHEMICALS
Galloylglucosides; minerals, protein, vitamins A, C, B1, B2; volatile oil (principally eugenol).

ACTIONS
Antioxidant, aromatic digestive, carminative.

INDICATIONS
Internally Dyspepsia, flatulence.

PREPARATIONS
Internally The fruits can be used as a condiment as part of the diet or prepared as a decoction or tincture.

CAUTIONS
None found.

Pinus sylvestris

COMMON NAME Scots pine.
PLANT FAMILY Pinaceae.

RELATED SPECIES There are around 100 species of pine tree, many of which are used medicinally including *P. palustris* (pitch pine). *Abies* (fir) species and *Tsuga* (hemlocks) species are closely related members of the Pinaceae.

RANGE Mostly northern temperate region in Europe and America.

PARTS USED Bark, volatile oil distilled from the leaves (needles).

OVERVIEW
There are many species of pine tree, most of which yield antiseptic tars. The wood of pines provides turpentine for paints and varnishes and is widely used for construction work, furniture making, railway sleepers and telegraph poles. The volatile oil is often used in cosmetics particularly in men's perfumes due to its perceived rugged, masculine scent. Constituents called oligomeric proanthocyanidins (OPCs, also known as pycnogenol) can be extracted from certain pine species. These have a supportive effect on collagen in the body's tissues and can be helpful to treat bruising and varicose veins. They also protect against cell damage (which can give a role in cancer prevention) and the build-up of fats in

the arteries (which can help prevent heart disease). Commercial OPC supplements are available made from the maritime pine (*P. pinaster*). Pine volatile oil is an excellent antiseptic for many kinds of respiratory disorders and is particularly helpful used as an inhalation for blocked sinuses, where it combines well with eucalyptus oil. Scots pine has been shown to inhibit the bacteria *Staphylococcus aureus*, which is resistant to many conventional antibiotic drugs.

Treatment tip – Bath oil

Pine oil can be added to baths where it is wonderfully penetrating and relaxing helping to release muscular tension. Add 10 drops of pine oil to 5ml of sweet almond oil and pour into the bath as it is filling. Due to their warming effect on the circulation pine baths are particularly pleasant taken in cold weather. Pine has a stimulating effect on the circulation as a whole, improving energy and mental functioning, so it is best to take a pine bath early in the evening not just before bed.

PHYTOCHEMICALS
Flavonols (oligomeric proanthocyanidins), volatile oil (including pinenes).

ACTIONS
Antibacterial, antioxidant, antiseptic,

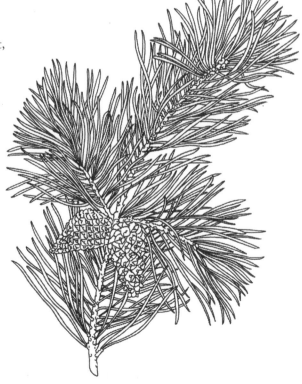

expectorant.
INDICATIONS
Internally Coughs and chest congestion.
Externally Respiratory disorders such as chest infections, coughs, sinusitis. Muscle disorders such as muscle stiffness and rheumatism.

PREPARATIONS
Internally Bark and leaf decoctions as well as the volatile oil itself have been used as ingredients in cough syrups. Pine flowers are boiled to make one of the Bach Flower Remedies; this is used to treat 'those who blame themselves'.
Externally The volatile oil is taken by inhalation or massaged into aching muscles diluted in a carrier oil. Bark or leaf decoctions can be added to baths, as well as the volatile oil.

CAUTIONS
Avoid undiluted volatile oils coming into direct contact with the skin. Wash your hands after handling volatile oils.

Piscidia erythrina

(also known as *P. piscipula*)
COMMON NAME Jamaica dogwood.
PLANT FAMILY Leguminosae.

RANGE Florida, West Indies.

PART USED Bark.

OVERVIEW
Jamaica dogwood is a deciduous tree growing in southern parts of North America and in the West Indies. The botanical name of this tree derives from *piscis* (fish) and *caedare* (to kill). This refers to the traditional practice of using the leaves and branches to make a fish poison. The preparation stuns fish, sedating them and making them easier to catch. Despite this, Jamaica dogwood is quite safe for human beings. It is a very useful treatment for anxiety-related problems. Taken on going to bed it helps to relieve insomnia and it is calming to people who are tense and overactive. For women it can help reduce period pain due to its muscle relaxing effects. It has traditionally been used to prevent miscarriage (only when miscarriage is threatened, not through the whole of pregnancy) and to treat labour pain and the discomfort following birth.

Treatment tip – Insomnia

Take 5–10ml of Piscidia tincture in half a glass of warm water on going to bed. It is generally helpful in insomnia to exercise more during the day time, eat regularly and healthily, and go for a good brisk walk followed by a warm bath before going to bed.

PHYTOCHEMICALS
Isoflavones, tannins, saponin glycoside.

ACTIONS
Analgesic, anti-inflammatory, antispasmodic, sedative.

INDICATIONS
Internally Anxiety, asthma, hyperactivity, insomnia, muscular pain (such as lower back pain), neuralgias, period pain, tension headache.

PREPARATIONS
Internally The bark is taken by mouth as a decoction or tincture.

CAUTIONS
Jamaica dogwood should only be used in pregnancy on expert professional advice.

Pistacia lentiscus

COMMON NAME Mastic.
PLANT FAMILY Anacardiaceae.

RELATED SPECIES *P. terebinthus* (terebinth tree).

RANGE The Mediterranean.

PART USED Mastic (resinous exudate from the stem).

OVERVIEW
Mastic is a small evergreen tree whose bark, when pierced, produces a sticky resinous substance, also known as mastic. This was traditionally chewed to treat bad breath and to plug dental caries (it is a hard concrete resinous substance). Recently it has been shown to kill the bacteria (*Helicobacter pylori*) associated with the development of stomach and duodenal ulcers. This may lead to it being used more widely for these problems.

PHYTOCHEMICALS
Resins, volatile oil (including pinene).

ACTIONS
Antibacterial.

INDICATIONS
Internally Possible treatment for peptic ulcers (stomach and duodenal ulcers).
Externally Bad breath, boils, ringworm, skin infections.

PREPARATIONS
Internally Mastic can be taken as a powder or tincture by mouth.
Externally Chewed for bad breath and applied as a lotion for other purposes.

CAUTIONS
None found.

Populus x candicans

(also known as *P.* x *gileadensis*).
COMMON NAMES Balm of Gilead; Ontario poplar.
PLANT FAMILY Salicaceae.

RELATED SPECIES see *Populus* species. Other *Populus* species whose buds are used in similar ways to those described include *P. balsamifera* and *P. nigra*.

NOT TO BE CONFUSED WITH Several other trees are known as Balm of Gilead including *Commiphora gileadensis* and *Liquidambar orientalis*.

RANGE North America.

PART USED Leaf buds.

OVERVIEW
The botanical origins of this tree are obscure and controversial, add to this the fact that its common name of Balm of Gilead is attributed to many other plants then it is not surprising that a lot of confusion surrounds this particular tree. The Ontario poplar produces extremely sticky leaf buds. This stickiness is due to a resin that is chemically similar to propolis produced by bees. The resin is so strong that it can cause burning of the lining of the mouth and oesophagus if you take poplar bud preparations neat; always dilute the tincture with water.

PHYTOCHEMICALS
Flavonoids, phenolic glycosides (including salicin and populin), resins, volatile oil.

> ### *Treatment tip – Immune boosting*
>
> Like propolis the Ontario poplar resin is highly antiseptic and stimulates the immune system. It is particularly of value in cough syrups and for colds and chest infections. To boost the immune system in colds and flus take 10 drops of the tincture in a glass of fruit juice or warm water 3 times a day.

ACTIONS
Analgesic, antimicrobial, anti-inflammatory, antipyretic, expectorant, immunostimulant.

INDICATIONS
Internally Bronchitis, colds, coughs, infected sinusitis.
Externally Arthritis, infected skin disorders (including ringworm), laryngitis, rheumatism, muscle stiffness and pain.

PREPARATIONS
Internally The buds are given as a tincture or syrup.
Externally Creams or lotions containing poplar extracts are used. The tincture can be used as a gargle for laryngitis.

CAUTIONS
Poplar buds are very resinous and the tincture particularly is highly irritant to the skin and the lining of the mouth. Do not use the tincture undiluted either by mouth or on the skin.

Populus species

COMMON NAMES See under Species Used.
PLANT FAMILY Salicaceae.

SPECIES USED Several *Populus* species are used in medicine including *P. alba* (white poplar); *P. nigra* (black poplar); *P. tremula* (aspen); *P. tremuloides* (quaking aspen). Also related are *P.* x *candicans* (Balm of Gilead), *Salix alba*; *Salix nigra*.

RANGE Eurasia (*P. alba* and *P. nigra*); Eurasia, North Africa (*P. tremula*); North America and Canada (*P. tremuloides*).

PART USED Bark.

OVERVIEW

Poplar trees are deciduous and usually grow quite quickly making them extensively planted as shelter belts. Poplar leaves have long stalks and are very mobile in the wind leading to the use of common names like 'quaking' aspen and species names like '*tremula*'. White poplar has white downy undersides to its leaves and when the wind blows these are upturned to create a beautiful effect. I have grouped all of the above species together, as they are all used in similar ways medicinally. They are related to willow trees and like them they contain salicylates, which are anti-inflammatory. Poplar bark is useful for treating muscle and joint aches and pains, it is helpful in colds and other febrile infections and it can ease period pains. Quaking aspen was used widely by Native American tribes and for several other conditions beyond those mentioned here. The Apache and others even used the inner bark as a food, for themselves and their horses.

Flower remedy

Doctor Edward Bach noted the 'shakiness' of poplar leaves when creating his flower remedies and made a preparation of *Populus tremula* to treat 'vague unknown fears'.

PHYTOCHEMICALS

Phenolic glycosides (including salicin and populin), tannins.

ACTIONS

Anti-inflammatory, anodyne, astringent.

INDICATIONS

Internally Arthritis, fevers, period pains, rheumatism, urinary infections such as cystitis.

PREPARATIONS

Internally The bark is given as a tincture or a decoction.

CAUTIONS

None found.

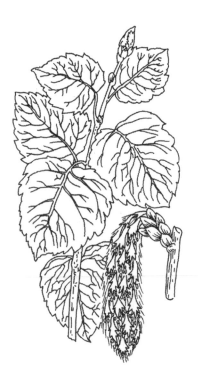

Prunus africana

(also known as *Pygeum africana*)
COMMON NAME Red stinkwood.
PLANT FAMILY Rosaceae.

RELATED SPECIES see *Prunus* species.

RANGE Tropical and South Africa.

PART USED Bark (from the stem).

OVERVIEW

Prunus africana is an evergreen tree that can grow up to 30m (100ft) tall and has small white flowers bearing small cherry-like fruits. The bark has traditionally been used for difficulties in passing urine. Research has shown that it benefits men suffering from enlargement of the prostate gland (benign prostatic hypertrophy – BPH). An enlarged prostate blocks the passage of urine and causes discomfort. This distressing problem is very common in older men. In BPH, testosterone accumulates in the prostate and is then turned into dihydrotestosterone, a potent form of testosterone that stimulates the gland to grow bigger. *Prunus africana* helps treat BPH in several ways:

- chemicals in the bark (phytosterols) compete with precursors of male hormones and prevent their build-up in the prostate;

- it reduces cholesterol levels in the prostate (this reduces male hormone generation because cholesterol is needed as a raw material to make the hormones);

- it reduces the level of the hormone prolactin, this has the result of decreasing the level of male hormones in the prostate;

- it lessens the degree of inflammation in the prostate.

A mixture of these actions helps clear the symptoms of prostate enlargement; it eases painful urination, reduces the frequency of passing water at night, improves sexual performance and helps to empty the bladder more efficiently and fully. It has also been shown to improve semen quantity and quality and may help in male infertility. The bark is safe and well tolerated but the demand for it has caused this tree to be classed as an endangered species. Unless it can be obtained from a guaranteed cultivated or ethically harvested source, a herbal substitute should be used such as saw palmetto berry or nettle root.

PHYTOCHEMICALS

Amygdalin, ferulic acid esters, phytosterols.

ACTIONS

Anti-inflammatory, anti-androgenic.

INDICATIONS
Internally Benign prostatic hypertrophy (BPH), impotence in men with benign prostatic hypertrophy or prostatitis, male infertility due to low sperm counts.

PREPARATIONS
Internally A bark decoction or tincture is used. Most of the research has been conducted on a special lipophilic (fat soluble) extract, this seems to be the most effective preparation and it is commercially available.

CAUTIONS
None found.

Prunus serotina

COMMON NAMES Wild cherry; American cherry; rum cherry.
PLANT FAMILY Rosaceae.

RELATED SPECIES see *Prunus* species.

RANGE East and North America.

PART USED Bark.

OVERVIEW
The bark of this American wild cherry is used to treat coughs. A pleasant tasting syrup can be prepared from it. This should be taken for the kind of cough that is dry and irritating and that doesn't bring up phlegm. The tree is also known as rum cherry because the distinctive taste of its bark has also been utilized in the making of rum and brandy. In North America the Cherokee used the bark for colds and fevers, the Chippewa found it good for worm infestation, wounds, cuts and burns and the Iroquois applied it as a poultice to the forehead and neck for headaches.

PHYTOCHEMICALS
Benzaldehyde, cyanogenetic glycoside (prunasin, this converts to hydrocyanic acid), tannins.

ACTIONS
Antitussive, astringent, sedative.

INDICATIONS
Internally Bronchitis, diarrhoea, non-productive irritable coughs, whooping cough.

> ### *Treatment tip – Coughs*
>
> For dry unproductive coughs take one teaspoon (5ml) of wild cherry syrup neat or in a little juice or warm water as required. You can take up to around 6–8 teaspoons a day. Children should take half that amount.

PREPARATIONS
Internally Decoction, syrup, tincture.

CAUTIONS
None found.

Prunus species

COMMON NAME see under Species Used.
PLANT FAMILY Rosaceae.

SPECIES USED *P. americana* (American plum); *P. armeniaca* (apricot); *P. avium* (sweet cherry, wild cherry, gean, mazzard); *P. dulcis* – also known as *P. amygdalus* – (almond); *P. domestica* (plum); *P. emarginata* (bitter cherry); *P. japonica* (Chinese plum); *P. mume* (Japanese apricot; wu mei); *P. persica* (peach); *P. spinosa* (blackthorn, sloe); *P. virginiana* and its varieties (chokecherries). See also, *P. africana* (red stinkwood) and *P. serotina* (wild cherry).

RANGE Prunus species grow throughout China, Europe, Japan and North America.

PARTS USED Bark, fruit, leaves, seeds and seed oil, depending on species.

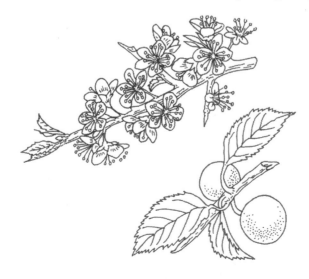

OVERVIEW

There are around 400 *Prunus* species, many of which are used as medicines. These species are grouped together because, while there are differences in uses, there are also many similarities. Essentially, most species contain the chemicals amygdalin and prunasin (particularly in the bark and seeds) which convert to hydrocyanic acid (prussic acid or cyanide). This chemical is safe in the small doses present in these trees and helps to alleviate coughs and other respiratory disorders. A synthetic version of this chemical (laetrile) was developed in the 1970s and was seen as a potential anticancer treatment as cancer cells are sensitive to cyanide. It proved to be ineffective but interest in cyanide for cancer has recently been rekindled with the use of immunologic markers to target cancer cells with cyanide while leaving normal cells untouched. This makes it possible to deliver a more effective dose to the cancer cells. Time will tell whether this new method works well enough to develop an effective anticancer drug. *Prunus* trees bear many of our most delicious and nutritious fruits such as apricots, cherries, peaches and plums. *P. dulcis* provides us with almonds and the oil expressed from this seed is the most commonly used type of massage oil. Other important massage oils include apricot and peach. Sloes, the astringent fruits of *P. spinosa*, are used to flavour gin. Branches of the American plum were used as sacred objects in the Sun Dance ceremony.

Flower remedy

Prunus cerasifera is one of the Bach Flower Remedies (cherry plum) used to treat 'fear of the mind being over-strained, of reason giving way, of doing fearful and dreaded things, not wished and known wrong, yet there comes the thought and impulse to do them'.

PHYTOCHEMICALS
Bark Cyanogenic glycosides.
Fruits Iron (apricots, cherries), complex sugars, malic acid.

ACTIONS
Anthelmintic (bark of American plum, fruits of Japanese apricot); astringent (most barks); laxative (fruits of the common plum); nutritive (fruits of apricot, cherries, peach, plums).

INDICATIONS
Internally Anaemia (apricots especially); asthma (twigs of American plum); constipation (plum); coughs (bark of American plum and others); diarrhoea (bark of most species, also the fruit stalks of sweet cherries were once used for this); for healthy hair, skin and nails, to promote optimal health as part of the diet and as a restorative in convalescence (the fruits and almonds); worm infesta-

tion (bark of American plum), parasite infestation (the fruit of the Japanese apricot).

Externally For poor skin tone, dry and aged skin (almond oil, apricot oil, peach kernel oil).

PREPARATIONS
Internally
Bark and leaves Decoction.
Fruits Eaten fresh or dried. For constipation dried plums (prunes) can be taken after soaking overnight in water, or they can be stewed, or the juice drunk.
Juice concentrate – The syrupy peach juice concentrate is an excellent flavouring for children's medicines.
Externally
Oil Several *Prunus* species yield fixed oils for use with massage and in cosmetic products. Apricot oil is prized for being light and easily absorbable.

CAUTIONS
Excessive eating of fruit can cause stomachaches and diarrhoea.

Psidium guajava

COMMON NAME Guava.
PLANT FAMILY Myrtaceae.

RELATED SPECIES *P. acutangulum*; *P. densiconum*; *P. guianense*.

RANGE Tropical America.

PARTS USED Bark, flowers, fruit, leaves.

OVERVIEW
This small tree usually grows between 5–10m (15–30 ft) in height. It bears large berries (yellow when ripe) the size of tennis balls, known as guava fruits. These delicious fruits are rich in vitamins A and C and are therefore an important nutritive. Guavas are up to 5 times richer in vitamin C than oranges. Several other parts of the tree have medicinal uses treating digestive, menstrual and other problems. In South Africa, where guava trees have become naturalized, the leaves are used to treat diabetes, fevers (including that of malaria),

coughs and wounds. Research has demonstrated that the leaves and bark are active against the amoebae that cause dysentery.

PHYTOCHEMCALS
Bark Tannins.
Fruits Pectin, vitamins A and C.
Leaves Glycoside (amritoside), volatile oil.

ACTIONS
Bark Astringent.
Flowers Menstrual agent.
Fruit Nutritive.
Leaves Astringent.

INDICATIONS
Internally
Bark Diarrhoea and dysentery.
Flowers Menstrual problems.
Fruits As a restorative aid in convalescence, bleeding gums.
Leaves Diarrhoea and dysentery, malaria.
Externally
Flowers Conjunctivitis.
Leaves Leucorrhoea (a white vaginal discharge), mouth ulcers.

PREPARATIONS
Internally
Bark Decoction.
Flowers Infusion.
Fruits Eaten fresh.
Leaves Infused.
Externally
Leaves Infused and used as a mouthwash or chewed for mouth ulcers. Infused and applied as a douche for leucorrhoea.
Flowers As a poultice for conjunctivitis.

CAUTIONS
None found.

Pterocarpus marsupium

COMMON NAMES Malabar kino; bastard teak.
PLANT FAMILY Leguminosae.

RELATED SPECIES *P. santalinus* (red sandalwood; red sanderswood).

NOT TO BE CONFUSED WITH The resinous compound from eucalyptus trees also called kino. Several other trees are described as kinos, due to exuding a similar material as *P. marsupium*.

RANGE India, Sri Lanka.

PART USED Gum exuded from trunk.

Conservation

Exploitation of *P. marsupium* for its timber and medicinal bark has lead to it being classed as being vulnerable to extinction in the wild in the medium term. *P. santalinus* faces extinction in the wild in the near future.

OVERVIEW
Malabar kino is a large deciduous tree with waxy leaves and grey bark. When the trunk is pierced a juice leaks out which dries into a gum. This is very astringent (tightens the skins membranes) and is used for diarrhoea and dysentery, mainly to stop the secretions of either. It also has a very important role to play in Indian medicine as a treatment for diabetes. Studies have shown that it seems to regenerate cells in the pancreas that are involved with sugar metabolism, making it a useful treatment for non-insulin-dependent diabetes. *P. santalinus* (known as red sandalwood though it has no relation to true sandal wood, *Santalum album*) is an important dye and an astringent used for dysentery and bleeding piles.

PHYTOCHEMICALS
Flavonoids, stilbenes, tannins.

ACTIONS
Antidiabetic, astringent.

INDICATIONS
Internally Diarrhoea and dysentery.
Externally Leucorrhoea (a white vaginal discharge), mouth ulcers, sore throats.

PREPARATIONS
Internally The powdered gum or tincture.

Externally A douche for leucorrhoea; gargle for sore throats; mouthwash for mouth ulcers.

CAUTIONS
This tree is not an alternative to insulin for insulin dependent diabetics.

Ptychopetalum olacoides

COMMON NAMES Muira puama; potency wood.
PLANT FAMILY Olacaceae.

RELATED SPECIES Several closely related species are also used in a similar way to *P. olacoides* including *Liriosma ovata* (also known as muira puama).

RANGE South America.

PARTS USED Bark, roots.

OVERVIEW
Muira puama is a small rainforest tree with flowers that smell of jasmine. It has a well-established reputation for supporting sexual activity. This accounts for one of its common names – potency wood. In men it seems to both increase sexual desire and improve difficulties in achieving and maintaining an erection. Interestingly, it has been used by South American tribes for preventing baldness. Although the mechanism for muira puama's effects is unknown, this use tends to support the theory that it has effects on reproductive hormones. Traditionally, its healing effects on neuromuscular problems are so esteemed that it has been used for paralysis.

PHYTOCHEMICALS
Alkaloids, phytosterols, volatile oil.

ACTIONS
Aphrodisiac, neurological stimulant.

INDICATIONS
Internally Impotence and sexual fatigue, rheumatism.
Externally Beri beri, neuromuscular disorders (such as neuralgias), rheumatism.

PREPARATIONS
Internally Decoction of bark and roots. It is thought that the constituents responsible for muira puama's actions are not easily dissolved in water so a long decoction (20–60 minutes) is required. It is likely that the tincture is the most effective preparation. Tablets are not likely to be very useful.

Externally Decoction of bark and roots (for 20–60 minutes) is used and added to baths or massaged into the affected parts of the body.

CAUTIONS
None found.

Punica granatum

COMMON NAME Pomegranate.
PLANT FAMILY Punicaceae.

RANGE South-east Europe to the Himalayas.

PARTS USED Bark, flowers, fruit (rind and seeds).

OVERVIEW
There are only two species in the pomegranate family, reflecting the uniqueness of this small tree. It is a beautiful plant with dark green shiny leaves and red waxy flowers. It is well-known for its fruit, which has an extraordinary interior architecture. It is full of seeds surrounded by an astringent tasting peel. The seeds are piled into interlocking pyramids and each individual seed has its own succulent and translucent covering. The seed pulp tastes bittersweet. It is used to produce the syrup grenadine. The calyx (the remnants of the flower left at the base of the fruit) is said to have provided the inspiration for the crown of King Solomon. Traditionally, it is seen as a symbol of female fertility. Besides being an important food substance pomegranate has mainly been used for tapeworm infestations. A preparation of the bark is taken to paralyze the worms followed by a strong laxative to remove them from the system. The fruit is particularly useful in the diet because it is quite bitter and has a stimulating effect on the liver, gallbladder and digestion. The fruit juice is a strong antioxidant, helping to support the health of the body's cells and reduce the risk of cancer and heart disease.

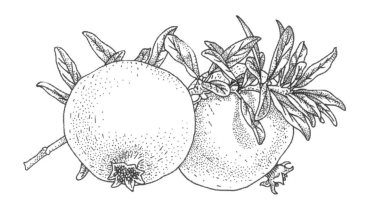

PHYTOCHEMICALS
Alkaloids, tannins.

ACTIONS
Bark Anthelmintic.
Fruit rind Astringent, bitter, aromatic digestive.
Seeds Antioxidant (seed oil), bitter (mild), demulcent, nutritive.

INDICATIONS
Internally Worm infestation (bark); diarrhoea and dysentery, fevers (fruit rind); as a restorative in convalescence (seeds).
Externally Fruit rind – leucorrhoea (vaginal discharge), sore throats.

PREPARATIONS
Internally
Bark Decoction.
Fruit rind Decoction.
Fruit/seeds Eaten fresh.
Externally Fruit rind decocted and used as a gargle for sore throats and a douche for leucorrhoea.

CAUTIONS
The bark may cause nausea and vomiting and should only be taken on expert professional advice.

Quassia amara

(also known as *Simaruba amara*)
COMMON NAMES Surinam quassia wood, stave wood.
PLANT FAMILY Simaroubaceae.

RELATED SPECIES *Q. cedron* (cedron); *Q. indica*.

NOT TO BE CONFUSED WITH *Picrasma excelsa*, the common name of which is quassia.

RANGE Tropical America.

PARTS USED Bark mainly, but also roots and leaves.

OVERVIEW
Surinam quassia wood is used as an insecticide in flypaper. It tastes very bitter and stimulates the secretion of saliva and digestive juices. It is traditionally used to improve the appetite and help in digesting food, particularly during convales-

cence following illness. It can be useful for indigestion and where the digestive system is too relaxed and congested. Surinam quassia wood is used in a very similar way to its close relative *Picrasma excelsa* (quassia), being also helpful for infestation with worms and for head lice. It is also given for amoebic dysentery and malaria.

PHYTOCHEMICALS
Quassinoids.

ACTIONS
Anthelmintic, bitter, vermifuge.

INDICATIONS
Internally Constipation, dyspepsia, fevers, loss of appetite, malaria, threadworms.
Externally Head lice.

PREPARATIONS
Internally Decoction or tincture of bark.
Externally Decoction or tincture applied to treat head lice.

CAUTIONS
Drinking strong preparations of Surinam quassia has been known to cause nausea and vomiting.

Quercus robur

COMMON NAMES Oak; common oak; English oak; French oak.
PLANT FAMILY Fagaceae.

RELATED SPECIES *Q. infectoria* has been used medicinally. *Q. petraea* (sessile oak) has similar uses to *Q. robur*. Many *Quercus* species have been used medicinally by Native American tribes including *Q. alba*; *Q. lobata*; *Q. rubra* and *Q. velutina*. *Q. suber* (the cork oak) has demonstrated anticancer activity in the laboratory.

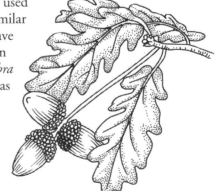

RANGE Europe, the Mediterranean.

PART USED Bark (from the young twigs).

OVERVIEW

There are around 600 different *Quercus* species (oak trees) and *Q. robur* is one of the better known. The oak is a mighty, large and long-lived tree with distinctive wavy-edged leaves and hard-shelled fruits (acorns). It grows throughout Europe but is particularly cherished in England where, for many, it is an evocative symbol of the country. Oak leaves used to be carved on British coinage and they form the logo for The National Trust, the UK's major conservator of land and historic properties. Acorns have been used as a food for pigs and as a coffee substitute. Oak bark is used for tanning leather. Ink can be made from oak galls (these are swollen balls created in response to parasite infection of the tree). Oak has been venerated as a sacred tree for many centuries throughout Europe and it continues to be revered today, partly for its great history and beauty, but also because of its vital role in supporting many hundreds of insects and animals, thereby contributing enormously towards maintaining a healthy countryside. In medicine its healing effects are due to the tannins that the bark contains, these are useful in treating diarrhoea, haemorrhoids and wounds.

Flower remedy

Oak is one of the Bach Flower Remedies, being given to 'support brave and strong people who never give up the fight, in connection with their health or everyday affairs, but who do not know how or when to give up and who have difficulty acknowledging their weaknesses'.

PHYTOCHEMICALS
Tannins.

ACTIONS
Astringent.

INDICATIONS
Internally Diarrhoea and dysentery.
Externally Haemorrhoids, mouth inflammations, nasal polyps, sore throats, wounds.

PREPARATIONS
Internally Decoctions or tinctures are used. A Bach Flower Remedy is available.
Externally Decoctions or tinctures are used as a mouthwash for mouth inflammations, or as a gargle for sore throats. It is used as a cream or ointment for haemorrhoids and the powdered bark is taken as a snuff for nasal polyps.

CAUTIONS
Oak bark is very highly astringent and can decrease the amount of nutrients absorbed from the diet. When taken internally (for diarrhoea) it should only be used for 3 or 4 days at most.

Quillaja saponaria

COMMON NAMES Quillaja; soap tree; Panama bark.
PLANT FAMILY Rosaceae.

RANGE Chile and Peru.

PART USED Bark.

OVERVIEW
Quillaja is an evergreen South American tree with attractive trails of waxy leaves. The bark is rich in saponins, which are soap-forming chemicals; the tree's name comes from quillai, a Chilean word meaning 'to wash'. The saponins are used to make ordinary soap and also as foaming agents in fire extinguishers. In medicine, saponins have the effect of helping to bring up mucus and catarrh from the chest in congested respiratory conditions. Quillaja is often used today as an ingredient in anti-dandruff shampoos.

PHYTOCHEMICALS
Saponins, tannins.

ACTIONS
Internally Anti-inflammatory, expectorant, immunostimulant.

INDICATIONS
Internally Chronic bronchitis, coughs.
Externally Dandruff.

PREPARATIONS
Internally Tincture.
Externally Shampoo with Quillaja extract is used for dandruff.

CAUTIONS
Quillaja may cause stomach irritation; internal use should be carefully monitored.

Ravensara aromatica

COMMON NAMES Ravensara; Madagascar cloves; Madagascar nutmeg.
PLANT FAMILY Lauraceae.

RANGE Madagascar.

PART USED Volatile oil extracted from leaves.

OVERVIEW

As the common names indicate, ravensara is one of the spice trees. Its seeds are used as spices in cooking and the bark has been used in making rum. Ravensara is gaining popularity today for the volatile oil distilled from its leaves. The oil smells like a cross between eucalyptus and tea tree and is antifungal and antibacterial, it has a relaxant effect on muscles and is slightly sedating. These latter qualities mean it is a good oil to use to help relieve muscular tension and aid sleep. It is also reputedly antiviral and is used on the skin to treat viral infections such as measles and shingles. It is a mild oil that is often well tolerated if used neat on the skin.

Treatment tip – Children's coughs and colds

Ravensara oil makes an excellent rub for coughs and colds in children. Mix 2ml (40 drops) of ravensara oil with 8ml (2 teaspoons) of a carrier oil such as sweet almond. Rub this over the child's sternum (breastbone), between the shoulder blades on the back and the soles of the feet. Doing this before bed-time will ease congestion and aid sleep.

PHYTOCHEMICALS

Volatile oil includes hydrocarbons (pinenes, sabinene), alcohols, oxides (1,8-cineole).

ACTIONS

Antimicrobial, anti-inflammatory, expectorant, nervine.

INDICATIONS

Externally
Volatile oil Colds, coughs, glandular fever, influenza, insomnia, measles, shingles.

PREPARATIONS

Externally The volatile oil is used as an inhalation or as a massage rub (diluted in a carrier oil or applied neat to small areas).

CAUTIONS

Although ravensara oil may often be well tolerated neat, it may cause sensitivity skin reactions in some people. It is best to test a drop of the oil on the skin before proceeding. Avoid using on the facial or genital areas.

Rhamnus species

COMMON NAME See under Species Used.
PLANT FAMILY Rhamnaceae.

SPECIES USED *R. cathartica* (common buckthorn; European buckthorn; purging buckthorn); *R. frangula* (alder buckthorn; black dogwood); *R. purshiana* (cascara sagrada; sacred bark).

NOT TO BE CONFUSED WITH *Alnus glutinosa* (common or black alder); *Hippophae rhamnoides* (sea buckthorn).

RANGE Eurasia (*R. cathartica* and *R. frangula*); the Mediterranean (*R. frangula*); North America (*R. purshiana*).

PARTS USED Bark (all 3 species), fruits (*R. cathartica* only).

OVERVIEW

These three Rhamnus species are all small trees. They are similar in appearance but alder buckthorn has red berries where those of cascara sagrada and common buckthorn are black. All are used as dyes and as sources for artist's pigments. The charcoal obtained from alder buckthorn was once popular in manufacturing gunpowder. All three species are laxatives. Cascara sagrada is considered a mild laxative, alder buckthorn is moderate and common buckthorn is very strong. Due to its severity, common buckthorn is generally no longer used; the two other species are to be preferred with cascara sagrada being the most widely applicable and popular. In all three types the fresh or young bark is very active and needs to be stored for 1–3 years before using. As it ages, the bark's effects become gentler and better to use. Emodin, one of the chemicals present in these trees has been shown to have antitumour effects and may yet have a role to play as part of cancer therapy.

PHYTOCHEMICALS

Anthroquinone glycosides (including emodin).

ACTIONS

Internally Bitter, laxative, cathartic, depurative, purgative.

> ### Treatment tip – Laxative
>
> For a laxative take 5ml of cascara sagrada tincture with the evening meal. In order to prevent any spasmodic abdominal discomfort, combine it with a carminative herb such as fennel (*Foeniculum vulgare*) or caraway (*Carum carvi*) to relax the digestive system. A mix of 5ml cascara sagrada with 5ml of caraway tincture in warm water is ideal.

INDICATIONS
Internally Constipation, loss of appetite, skin disorders such as acne and psoriasis.

PREPARATIONS
Internally Decoction or tincture of bark.

CAUTIONS
The young bark (under one year old) can cause abdominal pain, nausea and vomiting. Ensure only seasoned bark is used. *Rhamnus* species should only be used for short-term treatment. *R. cathartica* should be avoided.

Salix alba

COMMON NAME White willow.
PLANT FAMILY Salicaceae.

RELATED SPECIES There are around 400 *Salix* species. *S. caroliniana* (coastal plain willow); *S. fragilis* (crack willow); *S. humilis* (prairie willow); *S. mucronata* (Cape willow); *S. nigra* (black willow) and *S. purpurea* (purple willow) are among the many Salix species that have been used as medicines.

RANGE Eurasia, the Mediterranean.

PART USED Bark.

OVERVIEW
White willow is a tall, elegant deciduous tree. This versatile tree is used for basket making, and in the manufacture of Dutch clogs and cricket bats as well as being a source for medicines. Willow bark is well-known as a source of acetylsalicylic acid (aspirin) and, like aspirin, it is an anti-inflammatory. However, it does not share aspirin's side effect of tending to cause bleeding from the stomach. Willow does not contain exactly the same chemical as aspirin; instead it contains salicin which is converted by the digestive metabolism into salicylic acid and it is this

that causes willow's anti-inflammatory effect. Levels of salicin are generally higher in crack willow than white willow. Even so, the salicin content of willow trees is low and they cannot be considered as direct substitutes for aspirin. Willow preparations have a useful gentle ability to ease muscular and joint pains and to help control fevers. The American Eclectic physicians in the early twentieth century considered black willow (*S. nigra*) to have a particular sedative effect on the reproductive system, using it to dampen excessive sexual excitement in men and women.

PHYTOCHEMICALS

Flavonoids; phenolic glycosides including salicin and esters of salicylic acid; tannins.

ACTIONS

Internally Analgesic, anti-inflammatory, antipyretic, astringent.

INDICATIONS

Internally Arthritis, diarrhoea, fevers such as colds and influenza, gout, period pain, rheumatism and general muscular aches and pains including lower back pain.

PREPARATIONS

Internally Decoction or tincture of bark.

CAUTIONS

Willow bark is not a substitute for aspirin. If you are taking aspirin as an anticoagulant, to keep the blood thin, it is particularly important that you continue to use it, since willow does not have this property.

Sambucus nigra

COMMON NAME Elder; black elder; European elder.
PLANT FAMILY Caprifoliaceae.

RELATED SPECIES *S. canadensis* (American elder) has similar medicinal uses to *Sambucus nigra*.

RANGE Europe.

PARTS USED The flowers and berries are most frequently used today but the bark and leaves have also been used traditionally.

Treatment tip – Colds and flu

A traditional cold and flu treatment is made from elderflower mixed with equal parts of peppermint (*Mentha piperita*) and yarrow (*Achillea millefolium*). The mixture should be taken as a tea, drunk hot and frequently during the infection.

OVERVIEW

The elder tree is often encountered as a shrubby hedgerow tree but, given the opportunity, it can grow up to 10m (30ft) in height. It is one of the most revered trees in Western herbal medicine. This is partly due to its wide range of medicinal effects and partly because of the extensive folklore that has grown up around it. Until early in the twentieth century, hedge cutters would spare elder, out of respect for its supposed magical powers. The large creamy-white flowers smell of rotting flesh, this attracts flies for pollination purposes but also adds to the tree's mythology. Judas Iscariot is said to have hanged himself from an elder tree and legend has it that the cross of Crucifixion was made from elder. Anyone falling asleep under the tree was said to be transported to fairyland. Elderflower and elderberry have long been favourites of country wine makers. Medicinally the flowers and berries are used primarily for the treatment of colds and influenza. Elderflower cordial is a delicious way of enjoying the benefits of this marvellous tree. A study has found that an elder extract may play a role in treating diabetes, the authors noted that elder showed 'insulin-releasing and insulin-like activity'.

PHYTOCHEMICALS

Flowers Flavonoids, phenolic acids, triterpenes, volatile oils, fatty acids, tannin, mucilage, minerals (especially potassium).
Berries Flavonoids, anthocyanins, vitamins A and C.
Leaves Cyanogenic glycosides, flavonoids, sterols, triterpenes, tannins.
Bark Lectin, phytohaemagglutinin, triterpenoids.

ACTIONS
Flowers Antiallergic, anticatarrhal, anti-inflammatory, diaphoretic, diuretic, immunostimulant.
Berries Immunostimulant, laxative (mild), nutritive.
Leaves Laxative, purgative.
Bark Emetic, laxative.

INDICATIONS
Internally
Flowers
Arthritis – Anti-inflammatory; stimulates sweating and the passing of urine which assists in removing inflammatory waste products from around joints.
Catarrh – By improving the functioning of mucous membranes lining the ears, nose and throat they help clear catarrh in these areas.
Colds, influenza and other infections of the respiratory tract – Enhance the non-specific immune response, gently stimulate sweating in a fever, regulate temperature control and thus help to pass infections off more quickly and with less severe symptoms.
Hay fever – Combination of antiallergic, anti-inflammatory and mucous membrane soothing properties provide an excellent hay fever remedy.
Sinusitis, ear infections – Anti-inflammatory, immunostimulating and mucous membrane toning effects; antiallergic for year-round sinusitis (perennial rhinitis).

Berries
Cancer prevention – Anthocyanins have potent antioxidant effects.
Viral infections – Colds, influenza, viral infections of the upper respiratory tract.
Convalescence, debility, fatigue – The nutritional content can assist recovery and help improve energy levels.

Leaves
Bruises, sprains and chilblains, and wounds.

PREPARATIONS
Flowers
Tea For best effects drink as hot as possible, for colds and influenza drink frequently (up to about 6 cups a day), otherwise drink 2–4 cups a day. For a diuretic effect, the cold tea is thought to be more effective than the hot.
Tincture 1–5ml, three times a day, in warm water, between meals.
Cream Apply over maxillary sinus areas (on the cheeks just each side of the nose) to ease sinusitis.
Foot bath For night time coughs and fevers in children, use a foot bath before going to bed.
Eyewash For conjunctivitis. Apply twice a day (morning and evening) or as frequently as required.

Eye compress For tired or inflamed eyes. Apply lukewarm tea on cotton wool pads to the lids of closed eyes for 5–10 minutes as required.

Compress For chilblains. Apply to the chilblains for 5–10 minutes, 3–4 times a day.

Gargle For sore throats. Gargle for several minutes frequently until the soreness resolves.

Flower water Use neat for compresses, it has a cooling and soothing effect on the skin.

Berries

Juice 10mls, twice a day, in warm water, between meals.

Food Cook and sweeten with brown sugar ('elderberry rob') to make a nutritious and immune stimulating jam.

CAUTIONS

The flowers and berries are considered to be very gentle, safe and well tolerated.

Santalum album

COMMON NAME Sandalwood.
PLANT FAMILY Santalaceae.

RELATED SPECIES *S. spicatum* (Australian sandalwood).

RANGE India

PART USED Heartwood and the volatile oil distilled from it.

OVERVIEW

Sandalwood is a small delicate evergreen tree. It is semi-parasitic, relying partly on a host plant for some of its food. It is held as sacred by the Hindus, being a part of various rituals including funeral ceremonies. The wood is used in making cosmetics and perfumes. Sandalwood oil, the volatile oil made from the wood, is one of the most exquisite of all scents. It has a complex and sensual, warm and earthy fragrance. The oil is popular in aromatherapy where it is given for chest and urinary infections, skin problems, varicose veins and neuralgia. It has shown antiviral properties against herpes simplex viruses-1 and -2 (the viruses that cause cold sores and genital herpes). It is perhaps best known as a sexual tonic in cases of impotence and decreased libido.

It is known as a lover's oil, heightening the sexual experience when diffused as a room fragrance via an oil burner or applied as massage oil. Unfortunately, the oil is distilled from the heartwood of the tree and this makes it hard to harvest sustainably. It takes up to 20–40 years to grow a tree to the stage where it can be harvested. This has led to the tree becoming an endangered species so it cannot be recommended for use unless preparations are guaranteed as coming from an ethically harvested source.

Conservation

Sandalwood has been overexploited for its timber and oil and is now classed as being vulnerable to extinction in the wild in the medium term. Although it is illegal to export the timber from India it is being smuggled out of the country. A relative of sandalwood, *Santalum fernandezianum*, became extinct in 1908, harvested to death for its scented wood.

PHYTOCHEMICALS
Volatile oil Hydrocarbons (mainly santalenes), alcohols (mainly santalol).

ACTIONS
Analgesic, antispasmodic, antiseptic, antiviral, aromatic digestive, nervine, sexual tonic.

INDICATIONS
Internally Digestive disorders such as abdominal pain and indigestion; fevers; urinary tract infections such as cystitis.
Externally Cold sores, reduced libido and impotence, as a relaxant in stress and tension.

PREPARATIONS
Internally Decoction or tincture of heartwood.
Externally The volatile oil can be used as a room fragrance by diffusing in an aromatherpay oil burner, as an inhalation and as a massage oil (diluted in a carrier oil).

CAUTIONS
The oil is generally well tolerated when combined with a carrier oil and used externally but some people may be sensitive to it. It is best to patch test an area of skin with the diluted oil first.

Sassafras albidum

(also known as *S. officinale*)
COMMON NAME Sassafras; ague tree; cinnamon wood.
PLANT FAMILY Lauraceae.

NOT TO BE CONFUSED WITH A number of plants are known as sassafras because of a similarity in their smell (probably due to their containing safrole); they include *Atherosperma moschatus* (Australian sassafras) and *Doryphora sassafras* (New Caledonian sassafras).

RANGE North America and China.

PARTS USED Leaves; root bark and the volatile oil distilled from it.

OVERVIEW

Sassafras is a deciduous tree growing up to about 20m (70ft) in height with distinctive deeply-lobed leaves. The volatile oil was formerly used to flavour drinks including root beer. It was probably used in drinks partly for its taste and partly as a continuation of a tradition of using the plant to make a cleansing spring tonic drink. In the 1960s it was discovered that safrole, the chief chemical in the oil (up to 80–90% of the oil content), could cause liver damage and cancer. Use of the oil in foods and medicines is now banned or restricted in many countries. A safrole-free extract of the whole plant preparation is available but this has a question mark over its safety and besides, it is the safrole that accounts for most of the therapeutic properties of sassafras. The information in this profile is therefore for historical interest only; use of sassafras is not advised. In Native American medicine sassafras was an important medicine, being given for colds, diarrhoea, measles, rheumatism, skin diseases, worms, and wounds.

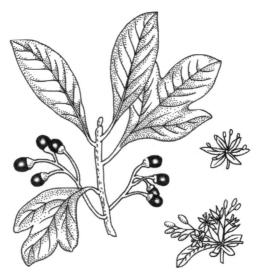

PHYTOCHEMICALS
Alkaloids (including boldine), resin, tannin, volatile oil (mainly safrole).

ACTIONS
Antirheumatic, antispetic, carminative, depurative, diaphoretic, diuretic.

INDICATIONS
Internally Colds and fevers, painful periods, rheumatism, skin disorders, syphilis.
Externally Abscesses and other skin disorders; abdominal and pelvic pain, bruises, rheumatism, sprains.

PREPARATIONS
Internally Decocted, or made by infusion (this retains more of the volatile oil content).
Externally Decoction or infusion of bark, applied in washes or poultices; volatile oil applied as a liniment.

CAUTIONS
Sassafras can damage the liver and is carcinogenic. It should not be used in any form.

Sorbus aucuparia

COMMON NAMES Rowan; mountain ash; quickbeam.
PLANT FAMILY Rosaceae.

RELATED SPECIES *S. americana* (American mountain ash); *S. aria* (whitebeam), *S. domestica* (service tree); *S. torminalis* (wild service tree).

RANGE Europe, South-west Asia.

PARTS USED Bark, fruit.

OVERVIEW
Rowan is a beautiful and elegant small tree with ash-like leaves and stunning clusters of berries that turn from yellow to orange to red as they mature. This is a truly lovely tree, each part has its own particular attraction from the intricate leaves and colourful berries to the slender stem and branches and the smooth pretty bark (the bark is especially attractive in younger trees). For these reasons it is widely grown as an ornamental tree in parks and gardens and as a street tree. It has long been seen as a sacred tree; thought to have the power to protect homes from harm it was often planted by houses. In Scotland, where it cuts a striking

figure against brooding autumn skies, it is particularly venerated and it is still thought to bring bad luck to fell a rowan, especially if it is near a house. The berries are stewed (with sugar, or sugar and apples) to make jellies and sauces and have been used in making beer and spirits. The berries have been used for their nutritive value (the berries of its related species, listed above, are also edible) but mainly they, and the bark, have been used as a treatment for their astringent properties in cases of diarrhoea and sore throats. In Native American medicine the Potawatomi used the leaves to make a tea to treat colds.

PHYTOCHEMICALS
Bark Tannins.
Fruit Fruit acids, sugars.

ACTIONS
Bark Astringent.
Fruit Astringent, nutritive.

INDICATIONS
Internally Diarrhoea.
Externally
Bark Leucorrhoea (vaginal discharge), sore throats.
Fruit Sore throats, tonsillitis.

PREPARATIONS
Internally Decoction or tincture of bark.
Externally
Bark Decoction given as a douche in leucorrhoea or as a gargle for sore throats.
Fruit Decoction as a gargle for sore throats and tonsillitis.

CAUTIONS
None found.

Strychnos nux-vomica

COMMON NAMES Nux-vomica; poison nut.
PLANT FAMILY Loganiaceae.

RELATED SPECIES *S. henningsii* (red bitterberry); *S. ignatii* (St Ignatius' bean); *S. minor* (snakewood). Many *Strychnos* species are climbing shrubs or lianas rather than trees.

RANGE India, southern Asia.

PART USED Seeds.

OVERVIEW

The sinisterly named *Strychnos nux-vomica* is an evergreen tree containing the potent alkaloid strychnine. Strychnine is highly toxic and can cause paralysis. It has a similar effect on the nervous system to tetanus toxin and causes lockjaw. Preparations of nux-vomica have been used as arrow poisons. In conventional medicine *Strychnos* alkaloids and their derivatives have been used in anaesthesiology. Recently they have shown some promise as antitumour medicines. In herbal medicine the tree has mainly been viewed as a bitter tonic to the digestive system and as a nervous stimulant in cases of fatigue and weakness. The American Eclectic physician Finley Ellingwood wrote, in 1919, 'wherever there has been depression or exhaustion of nerve force, it is the remedy'. In traditional Chinese medicine the seeds are said to 'unblock the channels' and are used for abscesses, swellings, pain following injuries and disorders of sensation such as numbness. The bark of the African species *S. henningsii* is used in South Africa for stomach problems and period pain; its unripe berries are taken for snakebites. Nux-vomica is one of the most important homeopathic remedies.

PHYTOCHEMICALS

Alkaloids (including strychnine).

ACTIONS

Bitter; stimulant (to the central nervous system); nerve tonic.

INDICATIONS

Internally Stomach complaints, tapeworm infestation, a restorative in debilitated conditions.
Externally Neuromuscular disorders.

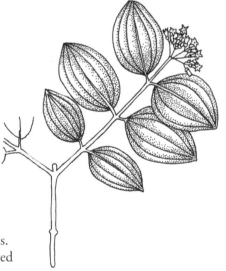

PREPARATIONS

Internally Pills, tinctures and decoctions.
Externally Paste made from the powdered seeds.

CAUTIONS

Nux-vomica can have powerful adverse effects on the nervous system, including causing spastic paralysis of the abdominal and chest muscles and the diaphragm, this makes breathing difficult and can prove fatal. Due to its toxicity it should not be used. The homeopathic preparation however does not contain any significant physical amounts of the plant and may be used without concern.

Styrax benzoin

COMMON NAMES Gum benzoin.
PLANT FAMILY Styracaceae.

RELATED SPECIES There are around 130 *Styrax* species, some of which are used as medicines including *S. japonicum*; *S. obasia*; *S. officinale* (storax); *S. tessmannii*.

NOT TO BE CONFUSED WITH *Liquidambar orientalis* (Levant storax) and *Liquidambar styraciflua* (sweet gum) both sometimes also referred to as styrax.

RANGE South-east Asia.

PART USED Resin extracted from stem.

OVERVIEW

Styrax benzoin is a small tree with fragrant white flowers. The resin exuded when the stem bark is incised is known as gum benzoin. It is a popular incense in India and is well-known as an ingredient of Friar's Balsam – a traditional inhalation for coughs and colds. Styrax resin is antiseptic and can be used to treat coughs and chest infections. In Ayurvedic medicine it is given for bedwetting in children. Tincture of benzoin is used as a preservative for fats and is added to medicinal creams to prevent them spoiling. The leaves of *Styrax tessmannii*, a related species, are used by several South American rainforest tribes to treat athlete's foot.

PHYTOCHEMICALS

Resin (including benzoic and cinnamic acids and benzaldehyde).

ACTIONS

Antiseptic, carminative, expectorant.

INDICATIONS

Internally Chest infections, coughs, urinary tract infections.
Externally Coughs, bronchitis, whooping cough (inhalation); mouth ulcers; skin infections and wounds.

PREPARATIONS

Internally As an ingredient in cough syrups as a tincture.
Externally Compound tincture of benzoin, or Friar's Balsam, is used as an inhalation. The tincture is diluted and applied to skin infections or taken as a mouthwash for mouth ulcers.

CAUTIONS

Resinous compounds can be irritating to the skin and digestive system; do not use Styrax tincture undiluted.

Syzygium aromaticum

(formerly named *Eugenia caryophyllus*)
COMMON NAME Clove tree.
PLANT FAMILY Myrtaceae.

RELATED SPECIES *S. cumini* (jambul; Java plum); *S. cordatum* (water berry); *S. gerardii* (forest waterwood).

RANGE The Moluccas.

PARTS USED Flower buds (the whole dried buds) and the volatile oil extracted from them.

OVERVIEW

The clove tree is a small evergreen tree. The history of the commerce in cloves is fascinating and often bloody. Growing originally only in a small region of the East Indies they were hard to obtain. The British, Dutch and Portuguese went to heroic lengths in order to pro-cure supplies of cloves, nutmeg and pepper, developing the lucrative but danger-ous spice trade. Cloves were seen as a culinary delicacy but were also used to treat disease. Pomanders (oranges studded with cloves) were thought to ward off the plague. Today, we particularly value the antiseptic qualities of nutmeg essential oil – it is still used in dental mouthwashes – but it is also relaxing and warming to the digestive system and relieves the pain of toothache. In toothache an infusion of cloves can be held in the mouth over the affected area. Drops of the essential oil in a carrier (such as olive oil) will have a temporary pain-relieving effect, acting as a local anaesthetic, and will help to subdue the problem until the cause can be found and treated. Cloves continue to be a culinary delight, used in many recipes such as apple pie and mulled wine. The bark of a related African species, *S. cordatum*, is taken to treat chest and stomach problems. *S. cumini*, known as jambul or Java plum, has been given for diarrhoea and diabetes (the fruit and seeds).

PHYTOCHEMICALS

Flavonoids, sterols, volatile oil (including mainly eugenol).

ACTIONS

Analgesic, anthelmintic, anti-inflammatory, antioxidant, antiseptic, aromatic, carminative, circulatory stimulant, expectorant.

Treatment tip – Colds and nausea

Infused clove buds (4–8 buds to a cup) make a lovely warming and aromatic tea for chills and colds, fighting infection and gently warming the circulation. Take this tea hot and sip it slowly, savouring the scent of the cloves as you do so. This can also be used for wet coughs, indigestion and nausea. Smelling the volatile oil can often relieve feelings of nausea as well.

INDICATIONS
Internally Chills and colds, coughs, indigestion, flatulence, nausea.
Externally Breath freshener, mouth infections, sore throat, toothache.

PREPARATIONS
Internally Infusion; tincture.
Externally Inhalation, or as a rub (diluted in a carrier oil). The infusion or tincture can be taken as a mouthwash for mouth infections and as a gargle for sore throats.

CAUTIONS
In toothache, cloves should never be used as a substitute for the attentions of a dentist.

Tabebuia impetiginosa

(also known as *T. avellanedae*)
COMMON NAMES Ipe roxo; LaPacho or lapacho; pau d'arco; taheebo.
PLANT FAMILY Bignoniaceae.

RELATED SPECIES There are around 100 *Tabebuia* species, many are used as sources of the medicinal bark.

RANGE Tropical America.

PARTS USED Principally the bark (especially the inner part), also leaves.

OVERVIEW
Tabebuia species are large trees with beautiful tubular flowers (the species with purple to pink flowers are thought to make better medicines than the yellow-flowered trees). They are highly valued for their timber; the wood is very hard and durable, being similar to mahogany. Most of the common names for the trees refer to their indigenous use for making hunting bows. Since the 1960s it has held a reputation as an anticancer treatment and more recently for treating

viral infections. Traditional and contemporary uses of pau d'arco cover a huge range of problems and this tree can come across as being something of a panacea. Its key property is that it enhances immune functioning and it is this central quality that accounts for much of its benefit. It is currently popular as a treatment for candidiasis and chronic fatigue syndrome. The potential of this fascinating tree is enormous – it could be of great value as a complementary treatment for cancer and leaukaemia, and help with the many viral and fungal infections that affect people with HIV and AIDS, as well as other immune system problems. It also appears to be a very safe and well tolerated remedy. Due to demand for timber and medicines many species of this wonderful tree are now endangered so ways to grow and harvest it sustainably must be found.

PHYTOCHEMICALS
Anthroquinones, flavonoids, nahpthoquinones (including lapachol).

ACTIONS
Antifungal, antiparasitic, antitumour, antiviral, depurative, immunostimulant.

INDICATIONS
Internally A supplementary treatment in cancer and leukaemia; candidiasis; chronic fatigue syndrome; fevers; opportunistic infections in HIV/AIDS; prostatitis; skin conditions (as below); viral infections such as herpes simplex (cold sores and genital herpes) and glandular fever (Epstein-Barr virus); weakened immunity.
Externally Skin conditions including eczema, infections (especially fungal such as ringworm), psoriasis, scabies, skin cancers; sore throats; thrush of the mouth or vagina; wounds.

PREPARATIONS
Internally Decoction; tincture.
Externally Decoction or a poultice applied to the skin, also as pau d'arco cream. The decoction or tincture is taken as a gargle for sore throats, a mouthwash for oral thrush and a douche for vaginal thrush.

CAUTIONS
Pau d'arco is not a replacement for conventional medical care in treating cancer. Surveys have shown that many pau d'arco products have low levels of the important chemical constituent lapacho, so it is important to use products of good quality.

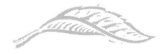

Tamarindus indica

COMMON NAMES Indian date; tamarind tree.
PLANT FAMILY Leguminosae.

RANGE Probably originated in Africa, now growing in India and throughout the tropics.

PARTS USED Bark, flowers, fruits, leaves.

OVERVIEW

The tamarind is an elegant and somewhat curious evergreen tree. It is in a genus of its own, having no closely related species, and it is unclear which region it originated from. It is tall and has wide spreading branches; these features have made it popular as a shade tree for which it is extensively planted. The fruits (tamarinds) are pods containing an aromatic sticky pulp in which the seeds are embedded. This pulp is reminiscent of dates and gives the name of the tree, 'tamar' meaning 'Indian date' in Arabic. Like dates themselves, the seed pulp is laxative. It is viewed as having a tonic effect on the liver, stomach and general digestion. It is given in convalescence as a nutritive and to promote recovery by engendering healthy digestive functioning and regular bowel movements. The fruits are also used in making sauces (including Worcestershire and HP sauce) and chutneys. The fruits are taken out of their shells and sold in compressed blocks. In India the leaves are boiled and given to children for worms. The bark is used for asthma.

PHYTOCHEMICALS

Plant acids, sugars, volatile oil (including geraniol, limonene, methyl salicylate).

ACTIONS

Flowers Anti-inflammatory.
Fruit Antiseptic, laxative, nutritive.
Leaves Anthelmintic.

INDICATIONS

Internally
Bark Asthma.
Fruit Constipation, fevers, poor digestive function.
Leaves Worm infestation.
Externally
Flowers Conjunctivitis.
Fruit Arthritis, ulcers, rheumatism.
Leaves Abscesses, arthritis, sore eyes, ulceration.

PREPARATIONS
Internally
Bark Decotion.
Fruits Eaten fresh or dried. An infusion can be made from the fruit pulp.
Leaves Decoction.
Externally
Flowers A poultice is applied over the eyes in conjunctivitis.
Fruit A pulp is made from the ripe fruit and a liniment is prepared from the dried fruit.
Leaves A leaf poultice is applied to swollen inflamed joints and abscesses.

CAUTIONS
None found.

Taxus baccata

COMMON NAMES Yew; English yew.
PLANT FAMILY Taxaceae.

RELATED SPECIES *Taxus brevifolia* (Pacific yew tree); *T. canadensis* (Canada yew); *T. cuspidata* (Japanese yew); *T. wallichiana*.

RANGE Europe, the Mediterranean.

PARTS USED Bark and leaves (needles).

OVERVIEW
This is a majestic and long-lived (up to 2,000 years or more) tree. It is viewed as a sacred tree, symbolizing both life (due to its great age) and death (due to its poisonous nature and dark, imposing stature). It is commonly planted in church-yards and other sacred places to represent this eternal duality. The wood is very hard yet quite elastic and was formerly used to make longbows for archers. Its main medical interest is as a source for the alkaloid taxol, which is used in con-ventional medicine to treat cancers, especially breast and ovarian cancer. Taxol is also obtained from other yew trees most notably the Pacific yew (*T. brevifolia*). Demand for taxol led to non-sustainable harvesting of the bark of this tree caus-ing it to become endangered. It has now been found that the needles of various yews will also yield taxol (though in smaller quantities than the bark) and pre-cursors of taxol. This is good news as needles can be harvested without killing the tree itself. Additionally it has been found that a fungus (*Taxomyces andreanae*) occurring on the Pacific yew produces taxol itself. The discovery that the hazel-nut tree (*Corylus avellana*) also contains taxol has raised hopes that it might be

obtainable from a variety of trees. Native American tribes used the Pacific yew for lung disorders and taxol is developing as a treatment for lung cancer.

PHYTOCHEMICALS
Alkaloids, diterpenes (especially taxol), lignans.

ACTIONS
Analgesic, antitumour, emmenagogue.

INDICATIONS
Internally Traditionally yew species have been taken for asthma, epilepsy, rheumatism, stomachaches, to bring on delayed periods and generally for pain.
Externally Traditionally for rheumatism and chest conditions.

PREPARATIONS
Internally Decoctions of the needles or twigs.
Externally The needles, boiled and the steam inhaled.

CAUTIONS
All parts of the yew tree are poisonous, except for the aril (the red part circling the fruit). Yew should never be taken as a herbal preparation. Its only place as a medicine is as a source of taxol in conventional chemotherapy.

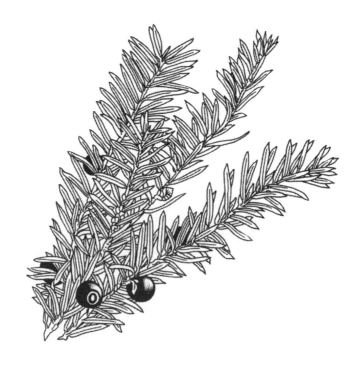

Terminalia arjuna

COMMON NAMES Arjun tree; arjuna myrobalan; kahu.
PLANT FAMILY Combretaceae.

RELATED SPECIES There are around 250 *Terminalia* species. Those used medicinally include – *T. bellirica* (beleric myrobalan); *T. catappa* (Indian almond); *T. chebula* (chebulic myrobalan); *T. sericea* (silver cluster-leaf).

RANGE India, Sri Lanka.

PARTS USED Principally the bark, the leaves to a lesser extent.

OVERVIEW

The name *Terminalia* is derived from the Latin terminus, 'end', due to the fact that these trees have their leaves gathered right at the very extremities of the branches, leaving much of the branch bare. *Terminalia arjuna*, the arjun tree, has been a major remedy in Ayurvedic medicine for at least 3,000 years. The bark is traditionally used for several types of heart problems including angina, endocarditis, pericarditis, and heart valve problems (weakness of the mitral valve). It appears to strengthen the heart's beating and to stabilize its rhythm. The bark is also used to treat bruises, fractures and when there is coughing of blood such as in tuberculosis. Studies have suggested that it reduces cholesterol levels and is a diuretic; these two qualities would also increase its effectiveness in treating heart disease, by reducing obstruction in the arteries and helping to remove the fluid that builds up (especially around the ankles) when the heart is failing. The leaves have been made into poultices for skin ulcers and sores. The fruits (called myrobalans) of two related species (*T. bellirica* and *T. chebula*) are dried and powdered and given to treat coughs, constipation and haemorrhoids. Another relative, *T. sericea*, is used in South Africa for diabetes, diarrhoea, pneumonia and stomach disorders.

PHYTOCHEMICALS

Flavonoids (including arjunone), phytosterols, tannins, triterpenoid saponins (including arjungenin), zinc.

ACTIONS

Antibacterial, cardioprotective, diuretic, hepatoprotective, possible hypocholesterolaemic.

INDICATIONS

Internally Angina, cirrhosis of the liver, coronary heart disease, congestive heart failure, diarrhoea, dysentery, heart arrythmias.

PREPARATIONS

Internally Decoction; tincture.

CAUTIONS

There have been conflicting reports about arjun's effects on blood coagulation and blood pressure, because of this and the serious nature of many of the problems it treats, it should only be used on expert professional advice.

Theobroma cacao

COMMON NAMES Cacao or cocoa tree; chocolate tree.
PLANT FAMILY Sterculiaceae.

NOT TO BE CONFUSED WITH *Erythroxylon coca*, the source of coca leaves and cocaine.

RANGE Tropical America.

PARTS USED Bark, leaves, seeds.

OVERVIEW

This is a well-known evergreen tropical tree whose fruits are large pods (which can be green, red or yellow) containing 20–60 cocoa 'beans' set in an edible white pulp. The seeds of the cocoa tree, when dried and roasted, are the source of one of the most highly-prized, not to mention delicious, tree products – chocolate. *Theobroma* translates as 'food of the gods'.

Although primarily seen as a confection, cocoa was formerly very important as a medicine and as a nutritive for building up sickly children in tropical America and Africa. It contains the stimulants caffeine (which is present in lower amounts than in coffee) and theobromine which was once used as a diuretic in conventional medicine, particularly in heart failure where it was frequently prescribed with *Digitalis* (foxglove). The leaves are used as a heart tonic in Colombia. The tree has been used since early times; evidence shows it being used by the ancient Aztecs and Mayans, who prized it so highly that the beans were used as a form of currency.

PHYTOCHEMICALS

Alkaloids – methylxanthines (caffeine, theobromine); fats; sugars.

ACTIONS

Bitter, heart stimulant, diuretic, nutritive.

INDICATIONS
Internally Formerly used as a diuretic, for heart conditions (leaves and seeds); and as a restorative agent in convalescence and weakness (seeds).
Externally Cocoa butter to soothe and nourish dry and chapped skin, and to soften the skin.

PREPARATIONS
Internally
Leaves Traditionally given by infusion.
Seeds Generally only taken as a food as solid chocolate and cocoa drinks.
Externally Cocoa butter is used as a carrier agent in making pessaries and suppositories because it can be made into a solid preparation but melts at body temperature. The butter is also used in cosmetic preparations such as skin creams.

CAUTIONS
Cocoa may trigger off migraine headaches. It should be avoided in all anxiety and hyperactivity disorders. Carob provides an alternative confection in these conditions – see *Ceratonia siliqua*.

Thuja occidentalis

COMMON NAMES Arbor-vitae; tree of life; Eastern white cedar.
PLANT FAMILY Cupressaceae.

RELATED SPECIES *T. orientalis* (Chinese arbor-vitae); *T. plicata* (western red cedar). *Cupressus* and *Juniperus* species belong to the same family.

NOT TO BE CONFUSED WITH Although commonly called Eastern white cedar, *Thuja* is not a member of the cedar family (*Pinaceae*).

RANGE Eastern North America.

PART USED Leaves.

OVERVIEW
Thuja occidentalis is an elegant conical-shaped evergreen conifer. It has scaly rather than needle leaves. Growing up to about 20m (65ft) in height, it is about a third of the height of its close relative *T. plicata*. Both are North American trees that have been used by Native American tribes. Several cultivars of each are grown as ornamentals. Arbor-vitae was traditionally used for colds, chest complaints such as pneumonia and tuberculosis, headache and toothache, rheumatism, skin problems and gynaecological conditions. *T. plicata* was given for a similarly wide range of problems. Arbor-vitae should be considered a potent

herbal medicine, for professional use only when taken by mouth, due to the high amount of thujone (a potentially toxic chemical) found in the volatile oil. However, when it is used with expert care it can bring pronounced therapeutic benefits. It has antitumour properties and is particularly indicated for female tumours particularly those that are benign (such as breast fibroadenomas and uterine fibroids) and also in some cases of malignancy (cervical cancer). It is antiviral and is active against human papillomavirus (HPV), which is associated with the development of cervical cancer.

Treatment tip – Warts and veruccas

The antiviral properties of arbor-vitae make it a useful external treatment for warts and verrucas. Surround the area of the wart or verruca with a little moisturising cream (to avoid the medicine touching normal skin) and paint a little neat tincture of arbor-vitae over the wart or verruca. Do this morning and evening for 2–3 weeks.

PHYTOCHEMICALS
Flavonoids, tannins, volatile oil (including ketones, especially thujone).

ACTIONS
Anthelmintic, antitumour, antifungal, antiviral, emmenagogue, expectorant.

INDICATIONS
Internally As a supplementary treatment in cancers including cervical cancer; amenorrhoea (absence of periods, but only when this is not due to pregnancy); cystitis; bronchitis and pneumonia; endometriosis; fibroids; viral hepatitis.
Externally Ringworm, skin tumours, verrucas, warts (including genital warts).

PREPARATIONS
Internally Decoction or tincture.
Externally The tincture or cream is used.

CAUTIONS
Thujone can stimulate menstrual bleeding and damage the nervous system. *Thuja* should not be taken at any time during pregnancy. It should only be used internally on expert professional advice. Even then it should not be given for extended periods of time.

Tilia species

COMMON NAME Lime trees; linden trees.
PLANT FAMILY Tiliaceae.

SPECIES USED *T. americana* (American lime, basswood); *T. cordata* (small-leaved lime); *T.* x *europaea* (common lime); *T. platyphyllos* (broad or large leaved lime).

NOT TO BE CONFUSED WITH Lime fruit comes from *Citrus aurantiifolia*.

RANGE Europe, Japan, North America.

PARTS USED Flowers with bracts (bracts are a leaf-like appendage to the flowers).

OVERVIEW

Lime trees are gentle and elegant, yet large and powerful deciduous trees with lovely heart-shaped leaves and pleasantly aromatic flowers. The scent of the flowers is said to have special properties; according to folklore those falling asleep under a lime tree could find themselves whisked away to fairyland. Honey from bees fed on lime flowers is thought to be amongst the finest of all honeys and is said to be calming and to help fight infections. Its pale wood is highly-prized and is used for making many things including musical instruments. The various species are difficult to tell apart. *T.* x *europaea* is a cross between *T. cordata* and *T. platyphyllos*. Linden tea is very popular in France, being used as a daily beverage. It has a honey-like taste and delicate aroma. Due to its sweet taste, linden tea is enjoyed by most children. This helps limeflower become one of the major children's remedies in herbal medicine. It helps to soothe irritable states, aid sleep, soothe coughs and clear colds. In adults it does the same things but can also be considered as a specific remedy to help protect the body from the effects of stress. It also boosts the immune system and helps to prevent heart disease (by reducing cholesterol levels and relaxing the arteries). It is also warming and relaxing to the digestive system, especially helpful for those of us who are frequently on the move and eating in a rush. If you are stressed, tense and overworked you need limeflowers! Three to four cups a day will keep the worst effects of a busy modern lifestyle away. The bark of *T. americana* was used by Native American tribes for stomach and urinary problems.

PHYTOCHEMICALS

Flavonoids, mucilage, phenolic acids, saponins, tannins, volatile oil.

ACTIONS

Antispasmodic, demulcent, diaphoretic, hypocholesterolaemic, hypotensive, nervine, sedative.

INDICATIONS

Internally Anxiety, insomnia, restlessness and irritability; catarrh; colds, coughs and fevers; headaches and migraines; high blood pressure and to help lower cholesterol; hyperactivity disorders in children; indigestion and irritable bowel syndrome; urinary infections.

Externally Agitation, hyperactivity, insomnia.

PREPARATIONS

Internally

Infusion – Limeflower tea is very pleasant, being aromatic, and tastes of honey.

Syrup – A syrup made for coughs and colds is particularly liked by children.

Tincture.

Externally

Footbath – For agitation, restlessness, insomnia especially in children.

CAUTIONS

Limeflowers can be sedating and should be avoided by people experiencing pronounced fatigue or they may increase the feelings of tiredness.

Treatment tip – Coughs, colds and flu

Throughout the time when coughs and colds are most prevalent, or during periods when you are under particular stress, take limeflower tea regularly. It can be sweetened with limeflower honey if you wish. For fevers in influenza take the tea made strong and drunk as hot as possible. A bath with limeflower tea added is also helpful.

Tsuga canadensis

(formerly named *Abies canadensis* and *Pinus canadensis*)
COMMON NAMES Canadian hemlock; eastern hemlock; hemlock spruce.
PLANT FAMILY Pinaceae.

RELATED SPECIES *T. heterophylla* (western hemlock); *T. mertensiana* (mountain hemlock). *Abies* and *Pinus* species are members of the same family.

NOT TO BE CONFUSED WITH The poisonous hemlock is a herb, not a tree, called *Conium maculatum*. Two related species are also known as hemlock: *Cicuta virosa* (water hemlock) and *Oenanthe crocata* (hemlock water dropwort). They are all members of the Umbelliferae family (fennel family) and completely unrelated to *Tsuga* species.

RANGE North America.

PARTS USED Bark, leaves (needles).

OVERVIEW
The eastern hemlock is a majestic large evergreen conifer capable of growing up to 50m (160ft) in its native region. *Tsuga* species are amongst the most beautiful of conifers, and many cultivars of eastern hemlock are grown as ornamentals in parks and gardens. Like other trees in the pine family, eastern hemlock contains a volatile oil that is antiseptic, stimulating and warming to the circulation. The needles are used to make both teas and external applications to treat arthritis and rheumatism. A steam bath was popular to relieve pain in arthritic joints and rheumatic muscles. This tree contains oligomeric procyanidins (OPCs) which act to prevent free radical damage to the body's cells and damage from fats. As a consequence they can have roles in preventing cancer and atherosclerosis (build-up of fat in the arteries leading to heart disease). The closely related western hemlock (*T. heterophylla*) has similar medicinal properties to eastern hemlock.

PHYTOCHEMICALS
Oligomeric procyanidins, resin, tannins, volatile oil (including pinene).

ACTIONS
Antioxidant, antiseptic, astringent, circulatory stimulant, diaphoretic.

INDICATIONS
Internally
Bark Colds, diarrhoea, urinary cystitis.
Needles Arthritis, colds, rheumatism.
Externally
Bark Laryngitis, mouth infections, wounds.
Needles Rheumatism.

Preparations

Internally

Bark Decoction or infusion of whole or inner bark for diarrhoea. Infusion of inner bark for colds and cystitis.

Needles Decoction or infusion.

Externally

Bark Decoction or tincture as a mouthwash for mouth infections and as a gargle for laryngitis. Pulped inner bark applied to wounds as a poultice to stop bleeding.

Needles Infusion or poultice applied to rheumatic areas. Leafy twigs were infused and the steam from this used for rheumatism.

Cautions

Eastern hemlock is rarely used at the present time. Internal use is not recommended. Most commercial OPC supplements are made from grape seeds (*Vitis vinifera*) or the maritime pine (*Pinus pinaster*).

Ulmus rubra

(also known as *Ulmus fulva*.)

Common names Slippery elm; red elm.

Plant family Ulmaceae.

Related species *U. americana* (American elm; white elm); *U. carpinifolia* (common field elm); *U. glabra* (wych elm; Scotch elm); *U. procera* (English elm). *U. procera* is one of the Bach Flower Remedies, used for those who 'feel that the task they have undertaken is too difficult'.

Not to be confused with *U. serotina* is also commonly known as red elm.

Range North America

Part used Inner bark.

Overview

The slippery elm tree is capable of growing up to 18–20m (60–70ft) high. The inner part of the bark is used in medicine; it is scraped off the outer bark and dried to a pink powder. This is one of the most mucilaginous of all plant substances. It was traditionally sold in two grades, coarse (for use as a bulking agent in other medical preparations such as poultices) and fine (for making soothing drinks). The powder swells up to make a gelatinous paste when mixed with water. It is very soothing and gentle when applied to the skin and was used as a base to which other herbs could be added in making poultices and other skin preparations. It is used as part of a 'drawing cream' applied to boils, stings, splinters and thorns. It helps to draw the infection or obstruction to the surface, removing it from the body. It is also used as a medicine in its own right, forming a soothing protective barrier over sore and inflamed areas of the skin and digestive system, allowing healing to take place. It is valuable in such problems as heartburn, stomach and duodenal ulcers and erosions, diverticulitis, sore throats. It also bulks and softens the stools making it valuable in constipation and to reduce irritation in haemorrhoids. It is also useful to take following food poisoning when it is hard to keep any other foods down and is good for sore, dry coughs and bronchitis. Slippery elm has long been promoted as a nutritive, restorative and strengthening food and is still sold as a beverage today. It is also a useful addition to cardiovascular diets aimed at reducing cholesterol levels since its mucilage content acts like soluble fibre in lowering the levels of fats in the blood.

Treatment tip – Heartburn

If you suffer from heartburn (*reflux oesophagitis*) take 2 slippery elm tablets, or 2 teaspoons of the powder mixed into a gruel, before each meal. Additionally, cut down your intake of fatty foods, take time to eat meals slowly, avoid orange juice and fizzy drinks and take up regular exercise.

PHYTOCHEMICALS
Mucilage.

ACTIONS
Demulcent, emollient, nutritive.

INDICATIONS
Internally As a restorative during convalescence and as a soothing nutritive and cholesterol lowering food for general use, particularly in the elderly. Digestive problems, including constipation, diverticulitis, dyspepsia, haemorrhoids, heartburn, inflammatory bowel disease (Crohn's disease and ulcerative colitis), irritable bowel syndrome (especially the type that involves constipation), stomach erosions, stomach and duodenal ulcers. Respiratory problems, bronchitis, dry cough.
Externally Abscesses, boils, swollen glands, sore throats.

PREPARATIONS
Internally
Powder The powdered bark is made into a gruel or drink by mixing one teaspoon with cold water then topping this up with hot water, stirring constantly so that the mixture doesn't go lumpy. As a restorative it is often flavoured with cinnamon or sweetened with honey.

Tablets Tablets are a convenient alternative to the powder. Take two tablets before meals.

Tincture Good quality tinctures are now available but are less mucilaginous than the powder.

Externally

The powder can be made into a poultice by adding a little water and mixing to a thick paste. The gruel can be gargled to soothe sore throats.

CAUTIONS

Slippery elm powder can be considered as a food. It is safe and well tolerated. The whole bark was once used to cause abortions by inserting the bark into the vagina as an irritant. The whole bark is still banned in many countries because of this. The powder, though, is entirely safe to take in pregnancy.

Viburnum prunifolium

COMMON NAMES Black haw; American sloe.
PLANT FAMILY Caprifoliaceae.

RELATED SPECIES There are around 150 *Viburnum* species. Amongst those used medicinally are *V. acerifolium* (arrowwood; mapleleaf viburnum); *V. lantana* (wayfaring tree); *V. lentago* (nannyberry); *V. opulus* (cramp bark), a shrub, this is an important species in herbal medicine being a major muscle relaxant.

RANGE North America.

PARTS USED Bark (of root and stem; some say that the root bark is more potent).

OVERVIEW

Many of the *Viburnum* species are shrubs rather than trees. They are often grown as ornamentals due to their showy clusters of flowers and often spectacularly colourful autumn foliage. Black haw is often encountered as a large shrub but it can grow into an attractive tree 6–9m (20–30ft) high. It has dark blue to black fruits ('black haws'), which are edible when cooked, and lovely red to yellow leaves in the autumn. The bark is used medicinally and it has traditionally been viewed as having an affinity for treating the uterus, having a relaxing effect on the uterine muscles. This means it is of help in a number of gynaecological conditions, especially period pain. Its calming and relaxant effects also make it of use in anxiety, insomnia and irritable states. A specific relaxant effect on the arteries means it can help to lower high blood pressure. The chemical constituent scopoletin is an antispasmodic for the uterus and salicin has pain-relieving properties. In Native American medicine it was seen as a tonic to strengthen the female reproductive system. It was taken both during pregnancy and childbirth.

The American Eclectic doctor Finley Ellingwood wrote that black haw was helpful in preventing repeated miscarriages. He says that it should be taken for around two weeks before the expected time of miscarriage (based on the time of the previous miscarriage/s) and continued for a week or two after that stage has ended. Black haw is also believed to be of benefit to relieve pain during childbirth, to prevent post-partum haemorrhage (bleeding following giving birth), to ease after pains and to assist the uterus to return to its pre-pregnant state. These are areas for expert attention and the plant should not be self-prescribed in these situations. In miscarriage, particularly, all attempts must be made to find and treat the cause before considering herbal medicine.

Treatment tip – Period pain

For period pain, black haw should be taken for a few days before the period is due to start and continued until the usual expected painful time (often the first two days of bleeding) has passed. Take 5ml in a little warm water twice a day and increase to four times a day if pain is present.

PHYTOCHEMICALS
Coumarins (including scopoletin), salicin, tannins, volatile oil.

ACTIONS
Antispasmodic, astringent, sedative.

INDICATIONS
Internally Anxiety, diarrhoea, heavy menstrual bleeding, high blood pressure, irregular periods, insomnia, period pain, threatened miscarriage.

PREPARATIONS
Internally Decoction. Tincture.

CAUTIONS
Black haw is not a substitute for conventional midwifery care in threatened miscarriage. It may be of value in recurrent miscarriage or in the latter stages of pregnancy when miscarriage is threatened by strong uterine spasms. It should only be used in these situations on expert professional advice.

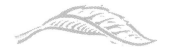

Virola species

COMMON NAMES Virola; cumala blanca.
PLANT FAMILY Myristicaceae.

SPECIES USED There are around 65 *Virola* species several of which are used for similar purposes including *V. albidiflora*; *V. calophylla*; *V. carinata*; *V. elongata*; *V. loratensis*; *V. surinamensis* and *V. theiodora*.

RANGE South America.

PARTS USED Bark (inner part), latex, leaves.

OVERVIEW
The bark of many of the small to medium-sized Virola trees is hallucinogenic. The main species used as an hallucinogen appears to be *Virola theiodora*, called oo-koo'-na by the Witoto tribe. Several other species are used for this purpose though. The bark is taken as part of shamanic ceremonies and as an aid to help the shaman (medicine man) contact the spirit world and diagnose disease. The inner part of the bark is prepared into a powder that is then taken as a snuff (often being blown into the shaman's nose by another person through a plant tube). Alternatively, the powder is made into pellets and taken by mouth by some South American tribes. Virola is in the nutmeg family and its fruits and seeds are very like nutmeg itself in appearance. They have a fleshy outer fruit containing a hard seed covered with a scribbly red membrane (called an aril). Beyond the hallucinogenic use there are more mundane applications for parts of this tree, particularly popular is the use of preparations externally to treat fungal skin infections.

PHYTOCHEMICALS
Bark Alkaloids; neolignans; tryptamines (these cause the hallucinogenic effects).

ACTIONS
Bark Psychoactive, antifungal, possible anti-inflammatory.

INDICATIONS
Internally
Bark As an aid to diagnosis in shamanic practices. For certain stomach and urinary problems.
Leaves Colic, dyspepsia, and it is given during childbirth to help progress when there are difficulties and to help induce labour when it is overdue.
Externally
Bark and leaves Applied to the skin for scabies and fungal infections.

PREPARATIONS

Internally Powdered inner bark taken by mouth as a pellet or as snuff. Bark and leaves have been infused to take as teas for digestive and urinary problems. Leaves decocted for difficulties in childbirth and to induce labour.

Internally Decoctions of leaves or bark and preparations of the latex applied to the skin for infections.

CAUTIONS

Virola is a potent hallucinogen and should not be taken internally. External use should be on expert professional advice only.

Vitex agnus-castus

COMMON NAMES Chaste tree; chasteberry; monk's pepper; agnus-castus.
PLANT FAMILY Verbenaceae.

RELATED SPECIES There are around 250 *Vitex* species. Several are used medicinally including – *V. negundo* (Chinese chaste tree); *V. rotundifolia*; *V. trifolia*. *V. agnus-castus* cv. *Alba*, is a white-flowered cultivar.

RANGE Southern Europe.

PART USED Fruits.

OVERVIEW

Vitex species range from tall trees to small shrubs. *Vitex agnus-castus*, though commonly known as chaste tree, is frequently encountered as a bush although it can grow as a small tree. It is deciduous and has spikes of aromatic lilac flowers that bear small fruits the size and appearance of peppercorns partly covered by a kind of grey velvety hood. The origins and meanings of the botanical and common names for this plant are open to debate. In Latin agnus means 'lamb', with agnus-castus meaning 'chaste lamb'. The tree has been associated with chastity for a long time. In men it certainly seems to have been used to suppress libido. It was taken as a condiment for this purpose in monasteries, to help the inhabitants preserve their vow of chastity, leading to the common name 'monk's pepper'. (Though it should be noted that chaste tree may improve male impotence if it is due to high prolactin levels). On the other hand Pomet, in his 'Histoire des Drogues' (1694), wrote: '… it is by way of Ridicule that the Name of Agnus Castus is now given to this seed, since it is commonly made use of in the Cure of Venereal Cases, or to assist those who have violated, instead of preserv'd their Chastity'. The major contribution of chaste tree as a medicine is its influence on reproductive hormones. It seems to act on the hypothalamus and pituitary gland, the 'control centres' for these hormones, rather than directly on reproductive organs such as the ovaries. The fruits inhibit the hormone prolactin and improve the balance between progesterone and oestrogen when progesterone levels are deficient. It has been helpful in some cases of infertility where there has been minor ovarian insufficiency (decreased progesterone levels) or high prolactin levels. It has a major use in treating premenstrual syndrome (PMS), especially where this involves symptoms such as bloating and tender breasts. It is less helpful where symptoms such as food cravings, headaches and dizziness are predominant. It is also valuable when the periods are irregular, too long or too short. It can be helpful for period pain except where the pain begins at the start of the period and is not preceded by PMS. It normally takes around 3 cycles for the benefits of chaste tree treatment for relief to become apparent. It is also helpful for women adjusting to coming off the contraceptive pill or hormone replacement therapy.

PHYTOCHEMICALS
Alkaloids (viticin), bitter principle (castine), flavonoids (including casticin), iridoid glycosides (including aucubin), volatile oil.

ACTIONS
Galactagogue, reproductive hormonal agent.

INDICATIONS
Internally Amenorrhoea (absence of menstrual periods, if due to high prolactin levels), acne (in men and women), benign breast disorders (fibroadenoma, cysts), endometriosis, heavy menstrual bleeding, infertility, irregular menstrual cycles, menopausal symptoms, period pain, postnatal depression, premenstrual breast pain and tenderness (mastalgia), premenstrual syndrome, prostate enlargement (benign prostatic hyperplasia), to improve milk supply in lactation (though this contradicts research showing that chaste tree decreases prolactin), uterine fibroids.

PREPARATIONS
Internally Decoction. Tincture. Chaste tree is usually taken in the mornings as it is thought that the pituitary gland is more active at this time and that the hormonal effects of the plant will therefore be more pronounced. The dosage for the tincture, for most of the above indications, is 5–20 drops of the 1:1 extract once a day. This may be higher in some cases on professional prescription.

CAUTIONS
Chaste tree is generally considered to be safe and well tolerated. Allergic reactions have been reported, such as skin rashes. Headaches and an increase in menstrual bleeding have been reported. Vitex should not be taken where there is uncomplicated spasmodic dysmenorrhoea (period pain occurring at the onset of bleeding,

not starting before or at the end of bleeding, which is not preceded by premenstrual symptoms such as breast tenderness). Women taking conventional hormonal drugs (such as the contraceptive pill, in vitro fertilisation treatment and hormone replacement therapy) should only take chaste tree on expert professional advice. It should be avoided during pregnancy.

Warburgia salutaris

COMMON NAMES Pepperbark tree; fever tree.
PLANT FAMILY Canellaceae.

NOT TO BE CONFUSED WITH Many trees are commonly called 'fever tree'.

RANGE Africa.

PARTS USED Leaves, stem bark, root bark.

Conservation

Pepperbark tree is now at high risk of becoming extinct in the wild in the near future. Attempts are being made to cultivate it in plantations.

OVERVIEW
This interesting tree grows in eastern parts of Africa with glossy leaves and round, green fruits. Its leaves smell of cloves and the bark is reminiscent of cinnamon. Leaves and bark taste of pepper and ginger. It is primarily used for colds, coughs and chest disorders but also for a wide range of other problems such as headache and toothache, malaria, rheumatism and skin complaints. It is also of importance as a 'magical medicine' to cure people who are bewitched. Due to its versatility as a medicine it is very popular and demand has now led to it becoming classed as an endangered species.

PHYTOCHEMICALS
Bark Drimane sesquiterpenoids (including warburganal), tannins.

ACTIONS
Bark Antibacterial, antifungal, aromatic digestive, bitter, expectorant.

INDICATIONS
Internally *Bark* For coughs, fevers, toothache.

PREPARATIONS
Internally
Bark The powdered bark is taken as a cold water infusion. It is also smoked for coughs and colds. The bark tincture is more antibacterial than bark infusions.

CAUTIONS
The pepperbark tree has not been extensively investigated but it contains very potent chemicals and should only be used on expert professional advice.

Zanthoxylum species

COMMON NAMES Common prickly ash, northern prickly ash, toothache tree (*Zanthoxylum americanum*); southern prickly ash, Hercules' club (*Zanthoxylum clava-herculis*).
PLANT FAMILY Rutaceae.

RELATED SPECIES *Z. bungeanum* (Chinese prickly ash); *Z. capense* (small knob-wood).

NOT TO BE CONFUSED WITH *Zanthoxylum* is sometimes spelt with an 'x' instead of a 'z', so *Xanthoxylum* is not a separate genera but the same thing. *Maclura tinctoria* is also known as toothache tree.

RANGE *Z. americanum* – East and northern USA. *Z. clava-herculis* – Central and southern USA.

PARTS USED Bark, fruits (berries).

OVERVIEW
There are around 250 *Zanthoxylum* species spread throughout Africa, America, Asia and Australia. The genus name *Zanthoxylum* derives from the Greek *xanthos*, 'yellow' and *xylon*, 'wood' because several species possess a distinctly yellow wood. This profile focuses on the two major North American species. Both are known as prickly ash, due to the presence of large thorns on their stems and branches and both have similar medicinal properties. They have been used to treat toothache and infectious disorders such as cholera and typhus (the alkaloid chelerythrine is antimicrobial). Their main attribute is that they stimulate and warm the general circulation, helping to improve oxygenation and nutrition of tissues and removal of the waste products of metabolism from the body. This makes *Zanthoxylum* species of particular value for arthritis and rheumatism and for peripheral circulatory diseases such as leg ulcers. This is how they are mainly employed in contemporary herbal medicine. Prickly ash can be useful if you suffer from poor general circulation, finding that you constantly have cold hands and feet. Various parts of the African species *Z. capense* (fever tree) are used for

abdominal pain, epilepsy, fevers and toothache. Chinese prickly ash (*Z. bungeanum*) is given in traditional Chinese medicine to 'warm the middle burner, disperse cold and alleviate pain'. It is used for abdominal pain and parasite infestation.

PHYTOCHEMICALS
Bark Alkaloids (including chelerythrine, fagarines, magnoflorine).

ACTIONS
Bark Analgesic, antimicrobial, circulatory stimulant, diaphoretic.
Berries Carminative.

INDICATIONS
Internally
Bark Arthritis, colds and coughs, fevers, leg ulcers, Raynaud's disease, rheumatism.
Berries Indigestion.
Externally
Bark Arthritis (painful, swollen joints) and rheumatism; sore throats; toothache; skin ulcers and wounds.

PREPARATIONS
Internally
Bark Infusion or decoction. Tincture.
Seeds Decoction and tincture.
Externally
Bark A poultice of the decocted root or stem bark, or pounded bark, was traditionally applied over painful teeth. Alternatively the tincture can be mixed into a paste with slippery elm (*Ulmus rubra*) powder and held in the mouth over the painful tooth. A decoction, poultice, tincture or cream is applied over affected areas for arthritis and rheumatism. Decoction or tincture as a gargle for sore throats.

CAUTIONS
Prickly ash can cause stomach irritation when taken by mouth; this can be avoided by taking it well diluted with warm water and after meals (within 30 minutes of eating). It may increase blood pressure so should not be taken if you have high blood pressure.

Ziziphus jujuba

COMMON NAMES Jujube; French jujube; Chinese date; da zao.
PLANT FAMILY Rhamnaceae.

NOT TO BE CONFUSED WITH *Ziziphus* is sometimes spelt *Zizyphus*.

RELATED SPECIES *Z. jujuba* var. *spinosa* (also known as *Z. spinosa*); *Z. mucronata* (buffalo thorn); *Z. spina-christi* (Christ's thorn).

RANGE South-east Europe to China.

PARTS USED Bark, fruits (jujube berries), seeds.

OVERVIEW

Jujube is a deciduous tree with yellowish flowers, it can grow to 10m (30ft) high. The fruits are edible but are more palatable when dried rather than fresh. They are dark red to black and look like small plums. In traditional Chinese medicine they are seen as a *qi* tonic. They strengthen the body, support weight gain, and enhance stamina and endurance. They are useful in weakened states including convalescence and chronic fatigue syndrome. There is some evidence to suggest they have an immune boosting effect. The fruits also help to soothe coughs, for which reason they were formerly much used in the West. The seeds of a variety of jujube (*Z. jujuba* var. *spinosa*) are used for their sedative properties in anxiety, irritability and insomnia. They are also helpful in reducing excessive sweating, especially night sweats. The bark of a common African species, *Ziziphus muronata*, is

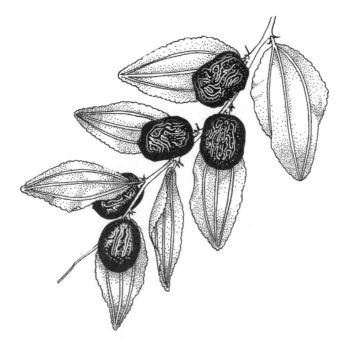

used to treat coughs and chest problems. Its leaves and roots are given to relieve pain. *Z. spina-christi*, a Mediterranean species, is said to be the tree that provided Christ's crown of thorns. *Z. mauritania* has been found by the National Cancer Institute to have an anticancer effect against melanoma (skin cancer) based on its content of betulinic acid.

PHYTOCHEMICALS
Fruit Calcium, flavonoids, iron, mucilage, saponins, sugars, vitamins A, B2, C.
Seeds (*Z. jujuba var spinosa*) – Saponins (jujubosides), volatile oil.

ACTIONS
Bark Astringent.
Fruit Antiallergic, antitussive, demulcent, hepatoprotective, laxative (mild), nutritive, sedative (mild).
Seeds (*Z. jujuba* var. *spinosa*) – anticonvulsant, hypotensive, hypnotic, sedative.

INDICATIONS
Internally
Bark Diarrhoea.
Fruits Constipation, coughs, debility and fatigue states, irritability, liver disease (hepatitis and cirrhosis).
Seeds (*Z. jujuba* var. *spinosa*) – anxiety, high blood pressure, insomnia, irritability, sweating (in anxiety, and night sweats).

PREPARATIONS
Internally
Bark Decoction.
Fruits The dried fruit is eaten.
Seeds (*Z. jujuba* var. *spinosa*) – Decoction.

CAUTIONS
In traditional Chinese medicine it is avoided in states where there is an excess of dampness such as in states causing bloating of the abdomen.

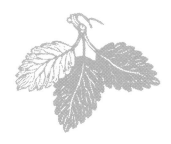

Glossary of Specialist Terms

Conventional medicine uses a lot of terms that are not in everyday use. Herbal medicine also has its own particular descriptive words that are not known to conventional medicine. A list of such words is given below. The main area in the book where these terms are used is in the 'actions' section of Part II, the tree profiles. I have included all the specialist herbal words used in the book plus an explanation of some conventional medical terms that sometimes cause confusion.

Abortifacient – A herb that may cause an abortion and therefore should not be taken in pregnancy.

Adaptogen – A substance helping the body respond to changing stresses and demands for example by improving physical and mental stamina and endurance.

Alterative – Alteratives restore healthy functioning of the circulation and lymphatic system, detoxifying the body and promoting healthy tissue growth.

Anaesthetic – Causing a loss of sensation. A local anaesthetic removes sensation to a specific area of the body. A general anaesthetic prevents sensations from being felt across the whole of the body.

Analgesic – Decreases sensitivity to pain without causing a loss of consciousness.

Anodyne – A medicine that takes away pain.

Anthelmintic – Herbs that destroy intestinal worm infestations. It has the same meaning as vermifuge.

Antiallergic – Substances that prevent or reduce allergic reactions.

Anticatarrhal – Substances that reduce the production of catarrh and the tendency to form phlegm/mucous.

Antihaemorrhagic – A medicine that stems internal bleeding.

Anti-inflammatory – A medicine that reduces the four cardinal signs of inflammation – redness, heat, swelling and pain.

Antilithic – An antilithic is a substance that prevents or reduces the development of stone formation in the kidney or gallbladder.

Antimicrobial – A substance that kills or inhibits the growth of infectious micro-organisms such as bacteria, fungi and viruses.

Antioxidant – A substance preventing free radical or oxidative damage to cells.

Antipyretic – A medicine that reduces fever.

Antiseptic – A substance that kills off infective organisms. The term usually applies to an agent that has this effect when applied externally to the body's surfaces.

Antispasmodic – A substance that relaxes muscles and thereby reduces spasmodic tension and pain. Spasmolytic has the same meaning.

Antitussive – An agent that reduces the tendency to cough.

Anxiolytic – A remedy that reduces the feeling of anxiety.

Aperient – This is a mild laxative. Usually plants have aperient effects by gently stimulating the production of bile from the gallbladder.

Aphrodisiac – A substance improving libido or sexual appetite.

Aromatic – Aromatics are plant constituents (usually based on volatile oils) that have an agreeable taste and smell. They tend to have a relaxing and warming effect. An example would be the use of cinnamon bark as an aromatic digestive – it improves circulation to, and relaxes the tissues of, the digestive system.

Astringent – A remedy that contracts tissues and thereby reduces secretions or excretions such as blood, mucous or faeces. Various astringents are useful to stop, for example, bleeding, over production of mucous or diarrhoea.

Bitter – A plant having a bitter taste. This usually has a stimulant effect on the digestive system including its associated organs such as the liver, gallbladder and pancreas.

Bronchodilator – A substance opening up the airways in the lungs. They can be useful in asthma for instance.

Cardioactive – A substance having an influence on heart functioning.

Carminative – Herbs that tend to relax the intestines. They can help reduce abdominal pain and flatulence.

Cathartic – A substance that causes marked movement of the bowels. It has a stronger action than a laxative.

Cholagogue – An agent that increases the production of bile in the gallbladder.

Cicatrizant – A substance that causes a wound to heal with scar formation.

Coagulant – A substance that promotes blood clotting. Can be useful in reducing bleeding.

Cytotoxic – An agent that kills specific body cells especially cancer cells.

Decongestant – A substance that reduces blockage and congestion in a particular area (for instance, a capillary decongestant relieves bruising; a nasal decongestant promotes a clear nose and improves breathing).

Demulcent – A herb that coats and soothes specific body linings. As an example – slippery elm powder makes a slimy gel that covers the linings of the oesophagus or stomach reducing inflammation in conditions such as heartburn. It is the internal version of an emollient.

Depurative – A substance that promotes detoxification. This term is particularly associated with plants that improve skin conditions by detoxification. Such herbs were formerly known as 'blood cleansers.'

Diaphoretic – A herb that increases perspiration. This can be important in the control of fevers and in detoxification via the skin.

Digestive – A herb that stimulates digestive functioning. (See also Aromatic and Bitter.)

Diuretic – A substance that causes an increased flow of urine.

Emetic – A substance that causes vomiting.

Emmenagogue – An agent that stimulates the menstrual period. Emmenagogues may often be abortifacients and should be avoided in pregnancy.

Emollient – This is a substance that has a soothing, softening and protective effect when applied to the skin. It is the external version of a demulcent.

Euphoric – A plant inducing a sense of extreme well-being. This sense may be excessive and inappropriate.

Evacuant – A substance causing a pronounced excretion of faeces.

Expectorant – This is a medicine that causes the bringing up of phlegm from the throat and lungs.

Febrifuge – A herb that reduces abnormally raised body temperatures. Reduces fevers.

Galactagogue – A substance that enhances the production of milk in lactating women.

Hallucinogenic – A substance that causes false sensory perceptions.

Hepatic – A substance that has an influence on the liver.

Hepatoprotective – A substance that protects the liver from damage.

Hypocholesterolaemic – An agent that lowers cholesterol levels.

Hypoglycaemic – A substance that lowers blood sugar levels.

Hypotensive – An agent that lowers blood pressure.

Immunostimulant – A substance that boosts the immune system improving our resistance to infection.

Laxative – An agent that promotes normal regular bowel movements. Used when there is constipation.

Nervine – A plant that has a beneficial effect on the nervous system. Nervines calm, nourish and strengthen nervous functioning.

Nutritive – A substance that has value as food for the body.

Oxytocic – A substance that stimulates contraction of the uterus. Herbs with this effect can be helpful in childbirth in trained hands.

Pectoral – A herb having an effect on the chest and lungs, such as an expectorant.

Purgative – Like a cathartic, a purgative is a substance having a very strong effect on promoting bowel movements. Purgatives need to be given with carminatives to prevent painful spasms occurring when they are administered.

Restorative – A herb that helps to restore normal functioning to a particular bodily organ or system.

Sedative – A substance that promotes calmness, and reduces excitability and tension. Sedatives may lower energy levels and reduce reaction times. Strong sedatives should not be taken when operating machinery, such as driving a car.

Spasmolytic – An agent that breaks down muscular spasm thereby relieving muscular tension and pain. Has the same meaning as antispasmodic.

Stimulant – A substance that increases the activity of a particular organ or body system. For example a cardiac stimulant increases the heart rate and force of heart contraction.

Tonic – A term applied to plants that have a supportive, enhancing effect on specific body organs or systems. For example a nerve tonic will strengthen and nourish the nervous system helping it to perform more effectively.

Trophorestorative – Plants in this category help to restore normal tone to body organs or systems. They typically help to restore optimal functioning where weakness has occurred. For example a venous trophorestorative such as horse chestnut helps to improve the tone of veins and it can therefore help in treating varicose veins.

Vermifuge – An agent that destroys worm infestations. It has the same meaning as anthelmintic.

Vulnerary – A substance that promotes the repair of wounds.

Bibliography

HISTORY

Cook, WMH, *The Physio-Medical Dispensatory*, WMH Cook 1869/Eclectic
 Medical Publications 1985
Ellingwood, F, *American Materia Medica, Therapeutics and Pharmacognosy*, Eclectic
 Medical Publications, 1919
Grieve, M, *A Modern Herbal*, Tiger, 1973 (first published in 1931)
Griggs, B, *New Green Pharmacy*, Vermillion, 1997
Hollman, A, *Plants in Cardiology*, British Medical Journal, 1992
Mabey, R, *Flora Britannica*, Sinclair-Stevenson, 1996
Milton, G, *Nathaniel's Nutmeg*, Sceptre, 1999
Minter, S, *The Apothecaries Garden: a history of Chelsea Physic Garden*, Sutton, 2000
Nadkarni, KM, *Indian Materia Medica* (third edition), Popular Prakashan, 1976
Porter, R, *The Greatest Benefit to Mankind: a medical history of humanity from
 antiquity to the present*, HarperCollins, 1997
Porter, R, Teich, M, *Drugs and Narcotics in History*, Cambridge, 1995
Rackham, O, *The History of the Countryside*, Dent, 1986
Tobyn, G, *Culpeper's Medicine: a practice of western holistic medicine*, Element, 1997

TREES

I consulted many books about tree details but the following require special
mention, I am indebted to their authors for the information they have provided.

Bean, WJ, *Trees and Shrubs Hardy in the British Isles* (Four Volumes), John Murray,
 1989
Mabberley, DJ, *The Plant Book*, Cambridge University Press, 1987
Thomas, P, *Trees: their natural history*, Cambridge, 2000

HERBAL MEDICINE

Bensky, D, Gamble, A, *Chinese Herbal Medicine: materia medica* (revised edition),
 Eastland Press, 1993
Bone, K, *Clinical Applications of Ayurvedic and Chinese Herbs*, Phytotherapy Press,
 1996
Bown, D, *Encyclopedia of Herbs and Their Uses*, Dorling Kindersley, 1995
Bradley, P, (ed), *British Herbal Compendium*, British Herbal Medicine Association,
 1992
Chevalier, A, *The Encyclopedia of Medicinal Plants*, Dorling Kindersley, 1996
Corrigan, D, *Ginkgo biloba: ancient medicine* (second edition), Amberwood, 1995
De Smet, PAGM, (et al), Adverse Effects of Herbal Drugs (3 volumes), Springer,
 1997

Ernst, E, (ed), *Herbal Medicine: a concise overview for professionals*, Butterworth Heinemann, 2000

Jones, K, *Pau d'Arco: immune power from the rain forest*, Healing Arts Press, 1995

Mills, S, Bone, K, *Principles and Practice of Phytotherapy: modern herbal medicine*, Churchill Livingstone, 2000

Murray, MT, *The Healing Power of Herbs*, Prima, 1995

National Research Council, *Neem: a tree for solving global problems*, National Academy Press, 1992

Pengelly, A, *The Constituents of Medicinal Plants* (second edition), Sunflower Herbals, 1997

Schulz, V, (et al), *Rational Phytotherapy* (third edition), Springer, 1998

Weiss, R, Fintelmann, V, *Herbal Medicine* (second edition), Thieme, 2000

Wehrbach, MR, Murray, MT, *Botanical Influences on Illness* (second edition), Third Line Press, 2000

Wren, RC, *Potter's New Cyclopaedia of Botanical Drugs and Preparations*, CW Daniel, 1988

ETHNOBOTANY

Arvigo, R, Balick, M, *Rainforest Remedies: one hundred healing herbs of Belize* (second edition), Lotus Press, 1998

Balick, M, Cox, P, *Plants, People and Culture: the science of ethnobotany*, Scientific American Library, 1997

Castner, JL, Timme, SL, Duke, JA, *A Field Guide to Medicinal and Useful Plants of the Upper Amazon*, Feline Press, 1998

Hatfield, G, *Country Remedies*, Boydell Press, 1994

Hutchings, A, *Zulu Medicinal Plants*, University of Natal Press, 1996

Moerman, DE, *Native American Ethnobotany*, Timber Press, 1998

Schultes, RE, Raffauf, RF, *The Healing Forest*, Dioscorides Press, 1990

Taylor, L, *Herbal Secrets of the Rainforest*, Prima, 1998

van Wyk, B, (et al), *Medicinal Plants of South Africa*, Briza, 1997

AROMATHERAPY

Penoel, D, Franchomme, P, *L'Aromatherapie exactement*, Roger Jollois, 1990

Price, S, Price, L, *Aromatherapy for Health Professionals*, Churchill Livingstone, 1995

Tisserand, R, Balacs, T, *Essential Oil Safety: a guide for health care professionals*, Churchill Livingstone, 1995

Valnet, J, *The Practice of Aromatherapy*, CW Daniel, 1982

Williams, DG, *The Chemistry of Essential Oils*, Micelle Press, 1996

NUTRITION

Ministry of Agriculture, Fisheries and Food, *Manual of Nutrition*, HMSO, 1995

Murray, MT, *Encyclopedia of Nutritional Supplements*, Prima, 1996

Phillips, R, *Wild Food*, Macmillan, 1994

Wehrbach, MR, *Nutritional Influences on Illness*, Keats, 1987

BIODIVERSITY AND CONSERVATION

Balick, M, Elisabetsky, E, Laird, SA (eds) *Medicinal Resources of the Tropical Forest: biodiversity and its importance for human health*, Columbia University Press, 1996

Grifo, F, Rosenthal, J, *Biodiversity and Human Health*, Island Press, 1997

Oldfield, S, Lusty, C, MacKinven, A, *The World List of Threatened Trees*, World Conservation Press, 1998

Walter, KS, Gillett, HJ, (eds), *1997 IUCN Red List of Threatened Plants*, IUCN, 1998

Wilson, EO, *The Diversity of Life*, Penguin, 1994

GENERAL

Barnard, J & M, *The Healing Herbs of Edward Bach*, Bach Educational Programme, 1988

British Medical Association and The Pharmaceutical Press, *British National Formulary*, BMA/TPS, 2000

Fortune, D, *Glastonbury, Avalon of the Heart, Aquarian*, 1986

Fulder, S, *The Handbook of Alternative and Complementary Medicine*, Oxford University Press, 1996

Frazer, JG, *The Golden Bough: a study in magic and religion*, Macmillan, 1983

Giono, J, *The Man Who Planted Trees*, Peter Owen, 1996 (first published 1954)

McLuhan, TC, *Touch the Earth: a self-portrait of Indian existence*, Abacus, 1982

Micozzi, MS, (ed), *Fundamentals of Complementary and Alternative Medicine*, Churchill Livingstone, 1996

Resources

CONSERVATION

There are, thankfully, many organizations involved in tree medicine related activities such as conservation work. In fact there are far too many to list! The selection below includes some of the most useful contacts but it is not exhaustive. Exploration of some of the websites listed below will generate a huge amount of links for you to explore further.

Australian National Botanic Gardens

Australia's premier botanic garden. The website provides some useful information about native aboriginal uses of trees for medicines. It also gives details of the Centre for Plant Biodiversity Research, a specialist centre for studying Australia's native flora.

GPO Box 1777, Canberra, ACT, 2601, Australia

Tel: (0061) 2 625 09450
www.anbg.gov.au/anbg/

APECA

The Association Promoting Education and Conservation in Amazonia focuses mainly on the conservation of the Peruvian Amazonian rainforest.

APECA, 12 South Main Street, Suite 302, West Hartford, CT 06107 USA

Fax/voice mail: (01) 860 232 6971
www.apeca.org

Carrifran Wildwood

A campaign for reforestation in the southern uplands of Scotland.

The Borders Forest Trust, Monteviot Nurseries, Ancrum, Jedburgh, Scotland TD8 6TU

Tel: 01835 830750
www.scotweb.co.uk/environment/wildwood/

Chelsea Physic Garden

Established by the Society of Apothecaries in 1673 this amazing place packs an astonishing array of medicinal plants into its 4 acres of walled garden and is active in conservation initiatives.

Chelsea Physic Garden, 66 Royal Hospital Road, London SW3 4HS

Tel: 020 7352 5646
Fax: 020 7376 3910
e-mail: enquiries@cpgarden.demon.co.uk
www.cpgarden.demon.co.uk/

CITES

Convention on International Trade in Endangered Species of Wild Fauna and Flora.
CITES is an international agreement which controls and monitors international trade in endangered species including medicinal plants.

CITES Secratariat, International Environment House, 15, Chemin des Anémones, CH-1219 Châtelaine, Geneva, Switzerland.

Tel: (0041) 22 917 8139/40
Fax: (0041) 22 797 3417
e-mail: cites@unep.ch
www.wcmc.org.uk/CITES/

Conservation International

An organization devoted to all conservation issues including protecting forests. It has a list of ethically produced, environmentally sustainable, forest produced foods.

Conservation International, 1919 M Street, NW Suite 600, Washington, DC 20036 USA

Tel: (001) 202 916 1000
www.conservation.org/

Ethnobotanical Resource Directory
The Resource Directory is on the web site of the Centre for International Ethnomedical Education and Research (CIEER). It provides access to everything that you could ever want to know about ethnobotany!

e-mail: info@cieer.org
www.cieer.org/directory.html

Ethnomedica
A project that aims to create an archive of British plant lore. Its main focus is on gathering accounts of traditional plant use from inhabitants of the British Isles.

Ethnomedica, Rhiannon Evans, 213 Broughton Road, Banbury, Oxon OX16 9RF

Friends of the Earth
Friends of the Earth and Friends of the Earth International campaign on the full range of environmental issues including conserving forests.

Friends of the Earth, 26–28 Underwood Street, London N1 7JQ

Tel: 0207 490 1555
Fax: 0207 490 0881
www.foe.co.uk

Future Forests
Provides the opportunity for individuals and organizations to become 'carbon neutral' by planting enough trees each year to offset our annual carbon dioxide production.

Future Forests, Hill House, Castle Cary, Somerset BA7 7JL

Tel: 01963 350 458
Fax: 01963 350 458
www.futureforests.com

Global Trees Campaign
This campaign is run by world experts in tree conservation. It aims to save the world's most threatened trees and their habitats through information, conservation and wise use.

UK
Global Trees Campaign, Fauna & Flora International, Great Eastern House, Tenison Road, Cambridge CB1 2DT

Tel: 01223 571000
e-mail: info@wcmc.org.uk

USA
Fauna & Flora International, 3490 California Street, Suite 201, San Francisco CA 94118

Tel: (001) 800 221 9524
Fax: (001) 415 346 7612
e-mail: faunaflora@earthlink.net
www.fauna-flora.org

Greenpeace
One of the oldest and most valuable of all conservation organizations. Greenpeace has an ongoing 'Amazon Campaign' to halt destructive and illegal logging in South America.

AUSTRALIA
Greenpeace Australia/Pacific, Level 4, 35–39 Liverpool Street, Sydney, NSW 2000

Tel: (0061) 2 9261 4666
Fax: (0061) 2 9261 4588
e-mail: greenpeace@au.greenpeace.org

NEW ZEALAND
Greenpeace New Zealand, 113 Valley
Road, Mount Eden, Auckland

Tel: (0064) 9 630 6317
Fax: (0064) 9 630 7121
e-mail:
greenpeace.newzealand@dialb.greenpeace.org

UK
Greenpeace UK, Canonbury Villas,
London N1 2PN

Tel: 020 7865 8100
Fax: 020 7865 8200
e-mail: info@uk.greenpeace.org
www.greenpeace.org.uk

**International Society for
Ethnopharmacology (ISE)**
This is a major scientific organization
dedicated to researching indigenous
plant medicines.

www.ethnopharmacology.org

Rainforest Action Network
RAN was set up to 'protect the Earth's
rainforests, and support the rights of
their inhabitants'.

RAN, 221 Pine Street Suite 500,
San Francisco, CA 94104 USA

Tel: (001) 415 398 4404
Fax: 415 398 2732
www.ran.org

Royal Botanic Garden, Edinburgh
One of the greatest botanic gardens in
the world; 'the Botanics' as it is known
to locals was established in the seventeenth century and now covers 31
hectares at its main site. It is involved
in a number of conservation projects
worldwide. One of its initiatives, Flora
Celtica, looks at the indigenous use of
medicinal plants in Scotland.

Royal Botanic Garden Edinburgh,
Inverleith Row, Edinburgh EH3 5LR

Tel: 0131 552 7171
Fax: 0131 248 2901
www.rbge.org.uk

Royal Botanic Gardens, Kew
England's leading botanic garden.

Royal Botanic Gardens, Kew,
Richmond, Surrey TW9 3AB

Tel: 020 8332 5000
Fax: 020 8332 5197
e-mail: info@rbgkew.org.uk
www.rbgkew.org.uk

Tree Aid
Promotes planting trees in Africa to
halt deforestation and soil erosion, and
provide food, fuel and incomes for
those in poverty.

Tree Aid, 28 Hobbs Lane, Bristol
BS1 5ED

Tel: 0117 934 9442

Trees for Life
Aims to regenerate the Caledonian
Forest in the Highlands of Scotland.

Trees for Life, The Park, Findhorn Bay,
Forres, Scotland, IV36 3TZ

Tel: 01309 691292
Fax: 01309 691 155
www.treesforlife.org.uk

Woodland Trust
Dedicated to protecting woodland in
the UK by purchasing woodland sites
and then caring for them in perpetuity.
They also replant lost woods and create
new woodlands. All of their forests are
managed in a way that benefits wildlife.

The Woodland Trust, Autumn Park,
Grantham, Lincolnshire NG31 6LL

Tel: 01476 581111
Fax: 01476 590 808
www.woodland-trust.org.uk

World Wide Fund for Nature

The WWF has an ongoing 'Forests for Life Campaign' that aims to promote forest conservation.

www.panda.org/forests4life/

MAGAZINES AND JOURNALS

British Journal of Phytotherapy

A journal for professional medical herbalists and interested members of the public.

The College of Phytotherapy, Bucksteep Manor, Bodle Street Green, Near Hailsham, East Sussex BN27 4RJ

Tel: 01323 834800

European Journal of Herbal Medicine

This is another professional journal that is also accessible to the interested non-professional reader.

The National Institute of Medical Herbalists, 56 Longbrook Street, Exeter, Devon EX4 6AH

HerbalGram

HerbalGram is the journal of the American Botanical Council and the Herb Research Foundation. It is an excellent and accessible source of information on herbal medicine both for the general and professional reader.

HerbalGram, The American Botanical Council, PO Box 144345, Austin, Texas, USA

www.herbalgram.org

Available in the UK from The Nutri Centre, 7 Park Crescent, London W1N 3HE.

Tel: 020 7323 2382
e-mail: enq@nutricentre.com

Journal of Ethnopharmacology

This is a specialist journal but it remains the pre-eminent resource for new research about plants from all around the world. It is produced by the International Society for Ethnopharmacology (see above).

www.elsevier.nl/locate/jethpharm

Reforesting Scotland

Developed as 'the tree planter's guide to the galaxy' and to support tree planting projects in Scotland specifically.

Reforesting Scotland, 62–66 Newhaven Road, Edinburgh EH6 5QB

Tel: 0131 554 4321
www.reforestingscotland.org

Resurgence

The leading forum for green ideas.

Resurgence, Ford House, Hartland, Bideford, Devon, EX39 6EE

Tel: 01237 441293
www.resurgence.org/
e-mail subscriptions: subs.resurge@virgin.net

HERBAL MEDICINE REGISTERS

American Herbalists Guild

Holds a list of approved herbal practitioners in the USA.

AHG, 1931 Gaddis Road, Canton GA 30115, USA

www.healthy.net/herbalists/

College of Practitioners of Phytotherapy

One of the major professional organizations for herbal medicine in the UK. Provides a list of qualified medical herbalists.

c/o College of Phytotherapy, Bucksteep Manor, Bodle Street Green, Near Hailsham, East Sussex BN27 4RJ

National Herbalists Association of Australia

The NHAA was founded in 1920 and provides details of qualified herbalists in Australia.

NHAA, PO Box 61, Broadway NSW 2007, Australia

www.nhaa.org.au

National Institute of Medical Herbalists

Established in 1864, this is the main professional body for medical herbalists in the UK. They can provide details of training courses in herbal medicine and a directory of qualified practitioners.

National Institute of Medical Herbalists, 56 Longbrook Street, Exeter, Devon EX4 6AH

Tel: 01392 426022
www.btinternet.com/~nimh/

SUPPLIERS

Healing Herbs

This company produces flower remedies made according to the original directions of Dr Edward Bach.

Healing Herbs Ltd. PO Box 65, Herefordshire HR2 OUW

Tel: 01873 890218
www.healing-herbs.co.uk

Organic Herb Trading Company

This company supplies medicinal herbs, tinctures and oils specializing in those that have been grown organically.

The Organic Herb Trading Company, Milverton, Somerset TA4 1NF

Tel: 01823 401205
www.organicherbtrading.com

Index of Common Tree Names

Note: page numbers in **bold** refer to the main entries for each species.

Index